Racing the Sunset

▾ ▾ ▾ ▾

Racing the Sunset
▼ ▼ ▼
AN ATHLETE'S QUEST FOR LIFE AFTER SPORT

Scott Tinley

THE LYONS PRESS

GUILFORD, CONNECTICUT
AN IMPRINT OF THE GLOBE PEQUOT PRESS

The Lyons Press is an imprint of The Globe Pequot Press

10 9 8 7 6 5 4 3 2 1

Printed in the United States of America

Library of Congress Cataloging-in-Publication Data

Tinley, Scott.
  Racing the sunset : an athlete's quest for life after sport / Scott Tinley.
      p. cm.
  ISBN 1-59228-095-1 (hard : alk. paper)
  1. Tinley, Scott. 2. Athletes--United States--Biography. 3. Athletes--Retirement. 4. Triathlon--Psychological aspects. I. Title.
  GV697.T56A3 2003
  796'.092--dc22

                                    2003017290

To all those who have been lost.
But mostly to those who were never found.

Contents

Prologue

"It was never that he was completely sold on athletic virtuosity as the be-all and end-all of problems; the trouble was that he could find nothing finer."

(From "Ring," an essay by F. Scott Fitzgerald)

*W*e sat in the tenth row. Well, more accurately, we inhabited the tenth row, for the present anyway. It was a gift, as all things of unencumbered beauty must be. "Here's a couple of tickets to the Stones concert. Have a nice time."

How appropriate, I thought, the Rolling Stones are old guys like me, reinventing themselves, part past, part future; trying to live in the moment because they had somehow come to realize that life was taking the moment away.

I glanced around the arena. As if it were just another real estate deal, the gray-haired pony tail set had laid claim to the memories of their youth. It wasn't that hard. At $300 for a decent seat, it only meant another billable hour or two, a small sacrifice to go back in time, back to when what you felt was raw, organic, before you made a distortion of your life, before you took the numbers 9–1–1 seriously. Before sex, drugs, and rock and roll became ears, nose, and throat.

To my far right I saw a friend: Janet, a fortyish personal trainer looking glorious in her new set of mostly exposed silicone twins, content in a marriage to a man who saw beauty below the reification. The 25-year-olds with chip-a-tooth-on-'em bodies had nothing on her. She seemed happy.

Up to my left I noticed another old bud, a tall man with a left foot welded in the shape of a 90-degree angle iron. Somehow, against all odds, he was swaying to the beat of Charlie Watts's percussion, perfectly. Their combined age reached three digits with ease. Then I remembered.

> **Me:** *"So, Bill...did you have any idea of what you were going to do when you left basketball?"*
> **Walton:** *"Not a clue. I had just had my ankle operated on. I'd never get to run a step again."*
> **Me:** *"Were you frightened, confused? I mean, it must have been quite disconcerting not having a future laid out in front of you."*
> **Walton:** *"Not really. I've always tried to look for the silver lining, all the good that's hidden inside of opportunity."*
> **Me:** *"So you..."*
> **Bill Walton** *says to me, as if he's discussing a new restaurant he likes:* *"I traveled a lot. Actually, I went on the road with the Grateful Dead for a year, just sat backstage and learned how to drum."*

I watched a 59-year-old Mick Jagger, reportedly logging 35 to 40 miles a week running, jump around the stage like a young Baryshnikov at an '80s disco. But for me, Walton was the show. A tented aloha print shirt draped around his graceful frame, he fit right in. I would've bought a magazine subscription from him if he came to the door one night or paid $500 to see him put up free throws at a Legend's game half time show. Bill Walton had reversed the oblique paradigm of time by insisting that it move through him instead of the other way around. Mick and Janet, same story. They had found their place by mocking time, then inviting it into their home.

Once you commit to a life of sport, you can never fully escape that part of your life. You can quit the game, pretend to play another, put on weight and say "all that" was in another life. But it wasn't. It's the same life, but you have simply learned to pretend better than most. You can fool the others; toss the pugmarks of your glory days into a dusty corner of the garage alongside a growing pile of rusty appreciation plaques. You can even play in the occasional master's event, hoist a few in the bar afterwards and talk about how the new crop of players just doesn't "get it." Much like doing jail time, it may grow quiet with the years, but hangs around your neck like a black crow or lyrics from the Eagle's *Hotel California*: "You can check out but you can never leave."

These things you do to create distance from what you once were and what you are now. These things you do out of fear. These things you do because you are both a former member of the entitled…and a survivor. Hard as you try though, you can never go far enough away.

It's almost embarrassing to say this, but I'm glad I'm not a professional athlete anymore. I know I was fortunate enough to take a moderate amount of innate talent, add years of incredibly hard work, mix in a dollop or two of luck, stir it well and bake it into the dream-come-true that so many young men and women fall asleep to at night. But as is the case with all dreams, they end in the morning. And while I enjoyed the heck out of that life, sports were but a long pause of what hopefully will be a much longer journey.

I won close to one hundred triathlons in my 25 year career, including the World Ironman Championships in Hawaii twice. But in the grander scheme of things that doesn't make me any better or worse as a person, as a human being. I could swim, ride, and run with the best of the world, but at times that made me a shitty husband and father. I could earn $10,000 for four hours work but that doesn't mean I would call up a friend on his or her birthday. I traveled the world on someone else's meal ticket, was given differed treatment at restaurants, border crossings, and dance clubs. Do I feel guilty about all that? Well, yes and no.

Professional athletes are revered in our society; right or wrong the faster you run or farther you can hit a ball with a stick, the more bennies that come your way. Triathlon doesn't even come close to the big time sports of basketball, baseball, football, or hockey. But I was given a glimpse of what it would be like to be a bona fide superstar, to be treated like royalty because of what you could do with your body and your mind. And while many would covet that life above all else, there are those who have been there and will tell you it's what you do with your heart, not your legs that matters most.

Okay, there are days I wish I could have earned enough money competing to retire on. But there are more days when I have to drag my sore back out of bed to go teach an 8:00 A.M. class in Creative Writing, and after a hot shower and cup of coffee, I say a silent prayer of thanks that I *have* to work, that I have purpose, a direction, a new skill and passion for something that needs me to have a good mind *and* a good heart to do the job well.

I shouldn't feel guilty for my athletic success. I worked damn hard for it. And in reality, I don't. But after the experience of coming down from that high perch of accomplishment, I know my training log needs to be filled with sentences like, "worked on being extra nice today" instead of "worked on being extra fast in the swim starts today." That's where the guilt comes in; I use it as a training tool to remind myself that I was very, very fortunate. And I damn well better not forget it, ever.

What I will never forget is the double-edged sword of great success. When I won a big race, the feeling was incomparable, heady, heady stuff. But I can also remember in the few hours of immediate celebration, actually feeling sorry for people who couldn't feel this way. How fucking arrogant is that? Why shouldn't a mother feel just as proud when her son comes home from school with a great report card or a business man facilitates a big deal that benefits all parties involved? You know where I might have been the luckiest in my career? It would be in having friends and family that kept me from thinking my shit didn't stink, that I was no different than any other man committed to his job, doing it well and proud of it. I won a lot of races, accountants crunch a lot of numbers, doctors treat patients, mailmen and women deliver a lot of letters. Life goes on.

But at some point it changes too. For an athlete the transition can be tough. But so can any of life's major shifts. People get old, accountants get fired, doctors make mistakes, mailmen and women have to retire too. We learn the most when we are thrown into a new fray, sometimes unprepared, always a bit nervous.

I thought my exit from sport would be easy. I had other things going, a clothing line with my name on it, a wife and kids, opportunities; I could not have been more wrong. Leaving sport kicked my ass.

But as I struggled to find a new identity, a new passion, a new place in the world, my personal growth went into overdrive. I might have learned more about myself and what's important in life in the two years after I retired than the previous twelve chasing that white line on the side of the road or that black one on the bottom of the pool.

To understand this, I had to go back and look at how I came to be an athlete in the first place; how we all come to be whatever we become. And I discovered this:

It gets inside you, slowly at first. You like the way it made you feel. Then you chased it hard, hunted it like a wounded animal. And finally, you let it in, fed it, watered it, watched it grow with pride and ego and continued to build it as you would restore an old car, knowing way down inside that you would never, ever be finished. And you didn't want to be. Couldn't allow it. For it defined you, this sport, this occupation, this career. Throw it away and just plain quit living. Simple as that.

> *"Imagine life conceived as a beautiful muscular organization—an arising, an effort, a good break, a sweat, a bath, a love, a sleep—imagine it achieved..."*
>
> (from Fitzgerald's "Ring")

The men and women who play sport all their lives, who make it a career, who get paid real money to put a ball through a hole, or run faster than the person running next to them, they are different. Some do it for the fulfillment of ego or to hear the crowd scream their name. Some do it for the money and a ticket out of a bad home, a bad 'hood. Some do it for loftier reasons, the love of the game, they will say, the raw pleasure of a solid hit or a personal best. And some of those athletes will truly mean it, or at least believe they mean it. Still others will commit themselves to a life of sport because they don't know what else to do.

The lure of the heroic athlete has a powerful force field around it. Sport gives them the opportunity to be a hero. Of course, so does walking downtown after dark, but a quarter million people won't witness you saving a homeless man from a mugging and walking him back to a shelter. There is always that chance though.

For every athlete who passes that gate though, the aura of hero becomes their identity, it validates their existence. Take it away and meet Mr. or Mrs. Vacuum.

I did it for all those reasons—or at least I knew that I could have. There *were* and *are* lots of reasons that I spent over half my life in a sport called triathlon. And as I grow older and continually redefine my involvement in sport, past, present, and future, I can't help but think it must be like a long-term marriage that endures separation, counseling, deep consideration, personal growth, and finally a kind of lasting reconciliation based on respect, acceptance, and appreciation.

Looking back at this exact moment in time, I realize the sport I chose had to have certain qualities: It had to be a tough one, just the right outlet for that obsessive-compulsive beast that lay inside. Perfect for exercising the demons of my past that fueled forty-hour training weeks and 20 races per season; the Lone Ranger on a titanium bike. I know I'll say it more than once between these covers—my sport had to allow me to be me.

An athlete thinks that he or she chooses which sport they will play, no matter if it's to lose 10 pounds on a bet with Larry in shipping and receiving or some game that gets under our skin and eventually becomes part of the flesh and blood that they are. But similar to choosing a mate, I think the sport chooses us. And we choose back in our mutual acceptance.

That's why there's always a price for all that we receive in return. The sport chooses and it sets the cost. Then, returning to our marriage metaphor, we must know that the commitment is a choice and if the costs outweigh the benefits, further choices of consequence must be addressed.

Driving through the neighborhoods, unconsciously peering into garages filled with dusty unused sporting goods, I have to wonder if those rusted stair-steppers and flattened basketballs are material evidence that the owners either got tired, lazy, re-directed, or simply re-prioritized their lives. In any case, there had to be a choice involved, and I for one would like any advance notice of a garage sale so that I too can fill up my garage with toys I don't have time to use, but if someday I make the choice to try something new, I can rest well knowing that I own a slightly used graphite tennis racquet or a pair of inline skates still in the box.

As I write these words, occasional drops of blood are falling on my keyboard. It's dark venous blood, not arterial and only one drip every minute or two. I can accept the mess, and I'm surprised at my patience. I wipe the drops off, first the *G* key and then right next to it, the *H*. I have to laugh because my tear ducts are so swollen they won't cry. Then I dab a not-so-sterile-anymore 4x4-inch pad on my nose again, wondering if blood is as bad as salty tears on a laptop.

I guess I should say, I dab where most of my nose used to be, a nice size chunk having been hacked off the day before, the victim of some skin cancer I can't pronounce.

The doc said it was the "good kind," which made me wonder if the bad kind would have required surrendering my cheeks, ears, and forehead; maybe my life insurance policy. And the surgeon, who I reminded to measure twice and cut once before he knocked me out to do his slice and dice thing, said that at least it looked like I had fun earning this operation.

A voice said: *Yeah, I had a hell of a good time swimming those 8 times 400 yard swim sets under the relentless southern California noon-time sun. Five or six days a week for almost 20 years. Great fun doc.*

Always a price.
But always a payday.

Halfway between remembering and imagining, I see myself sitting in the spa after those swim workouts, yakking away with my buddies, wondering if we should race in Mazatlan next weekend or just do the short race on Maui; thinking about whether we should have the turkey with avocado for lunch or just a couple of smoothies, knowing we'd be running later that afternoon. Not a care in the world, poking fun at the lawyers changing into their monkey suits in the locker room, a wad of fresh hundred dollar prize money bills in the back pockets of our baggy shorts...always as tan as a desert lizard.

The world had done its magic on us: we were immortal, we were athletes.

Somehow though, time had annulled a lot of that. The memories had grown opaque, softened with the years, left the building with Elvis. And I still had a few dozen years to fill up, a few kids to get through college, a few holes in my face. The sobering drift of things to come hit me like a wild throw from a control pitcher. I had to find work. I had to mow the lawn. I had to grow up. And someday, some asshole would tell me I was dying and there wasn't anything I could do about it.

No matter what the press says, there's never a precise moment when an athlete knows he or she has to retire. It's always a slow, painful bargaining, an Israeli taxi stand style of negotiating. Even for those who get hurt and the future comes up hard and fast and moves in like disease, there is always a period of negotiating.

Ok, you did some cool things, you were lucky.

Yeah, but maybe I'm not quite ready to go.

Hey, listen...no one is every *really* ready to leave. They just say stupid shit like, "I wanted to go out on top."

So...what will I do next? You don't expect me to, like, get a real job or anything, do you?

You've never been afraid of hard work before. Why the fear of a little sweat?

I'm not afraid of working, it's just that...

What? You just don't want to be like everybody else?

I guess that's part of it. For all these years I have slept the sleep of the gifted. I was somebody. I was in control.

An illusion little brother. You fancied yourself a rebel, telling the world to fuck off. What about that big sponsor logo on your chest?

What was that? Gang grafitti? Time to get real.

Ok, so send me to the school for normal people, tell me what textbooks to read.

It ain't that easy. It's called life. You missed that part while you were busy being "gifted." No make-up classes allowed.

So what you're telling me is that I can never be who I was again?

Just the opposite my newly humbled friend. You have to remember who you were, or more definitively, who you are. All that sport stuff was a fun job. You didn't really think it could turn into a career did you?

Actually some athletes do make a career out of what they did with a stick and a ball or a pair of ice skates or a titanium bicycle. And they are all too happy about it. But there is a fine line between the refusal to retire, to quit the game completely, and the decision to go on living. It's more about letting go than it is hanging on.

It's a complicated paradigm, a puzzle with many pieces. In rebuilding your life after sport, you have to find the straight edges and corners first before working towards the middle. The difficulty lies in the fact that your "middle" has been insulated for so long. As a star athlete, you aren't expected to do the little things like dealing with rental cars and paying power bills and managing your finances. Other people do that for you. They make sure your uniform is clean and your drink is full. You aren't expected to grow up because that would mean you're getting older, wiser. And slower.

And one day, you are slower; slow enough to be replaced. But you aren't necessarily wiser or more mature. The pieces of your life's puzzle are scattered on the floor of the locker you were just told to clean out to make room for "the new kid."

You may be very intelligent, very creative, you may have money in the bank and more friends than you can count. But you still have to stand naked to the world and decide what you're going to be when you grow up.

> *"…then imagine trying to apply this standard to the horribly complicated mess of living, where nothing, even the greatest conceptions and workings and achievements is nothing but messy, spotty and tortuous…"*
>
> (from Fitzgerald's "Ring")

That will be the hardest thing that most athletes will ever face, that need to mature from a teenager to a full grown man…when the mirror tells you that you are already 28 or 34 or 43. It is a compressed, turbulent period.

Decisions have to be made. You aren't trained in hard decisions. Most of those have been made for you.

It was a black-and-white world in which you lived. At the end of the day, at the end of the game or the race, you always knew where you stood. One NFL player, when asked what he missed the most, relied, "The scoreboard. I miss the scoreboard."

What he missed was the clarity of it all. He could look up at the scoreboard and it would tell him all that he needed to know.

In the real world of business or academia or life itself, the duplicity will eat a child alive. As an athlete, it takes a while to create a new type of score board. Some athletes never manage it. Others move seamlessly on to new playing fields. Most of them spend months or years building the new puzzle, one damn little piece at a time, wrestling with the pain of no identity every time they sit down at that table and see all those pieces of their life…scattered when it all used to be such a pretty picture.

After all that fame, so many athletes long to be just another regular guy—because regular guys don't have to carry the heavy burden of the hero. They don't have to sign autographs and dress well and say the right things and make the press happy. Yeah, after a few years in the tumult of total reification, normal seems pretty attractive.

Healing takes time. It takes work. Athletes aren't afraid of hard work, but they like to know how to train, and what they are working towards. Like hockey great Gordie Howe once said, "They teach you how to play the game but they don't teach you how to leave it."

"And then one can imagine the confusion that Ring faced on coming out of the park."

Truth be known, I wrote this as a form of healing; trying to understand the paradigm of lost identity, at the hands of a career ending young. It was the best training manual I could study, and the library was the best hospital I could check into.

I want others to know and heal themselves so that I too can be made whole again. I just want to be a regular guy again. Is that too much to ask? Is that even possible?

And if not, what are my chances of finding something that might even come close to allowing me some joy, fulfillment and purpose in what is left of my life? Right now I don't know. They say that a person is lucky to find one true thing in his life that he or she can become totally passionate about, a thing that challenges and heals and nurtures and rewards and kicks your ass and you love more than love—a thing that defines you, that gives you a reason for living.

Is it too much to ask for more than one of those things in a life?

I now stand alongside many others who have somehow achieved what they set out to do in their lives; they were successful, they made it—but they made it too soon. And then the troubles began.

A professional athlete's transition out of sport differs only slightly from the businessman selling the company he built, the mother sending a last child off to college or a career politician failing to get re-elected. For the athlete, it happens early, it can happen suddenly and unexpectedly. And it is compressed, tied to other psychological issues and more often than not, finds the athlete unprepared for a life beyond sport.

Today, things happen faster than they once did. And though we live longer, I'm not so sure the quality of life, even with our wondrous array of finger-tip conveniences, is better than our parents or grandparents.

Sport has become an integral part of every aspect of our society and our culture. With the media's help, sport has been woven deeply into our psyche. *This* period in time, not the Roman Empire, will historically be considered the "golden age of sport."

Do we not owe it to ourselves and those who we would let entertain us, who we would emulate, who we would worship as kings and queens, to look deeper at their lives beyond sport? For is not that an opportunity for us to look at ourselves and what we have or will face in the years to come?

Part One:

▼ ▼ ▼ ▼

"AND I'LL GET PAID FOR THIS?"

The Moment of Aloha

"The athletic realm involves the quest for being, realized through its fundamental mode of embodiment, the human body, and through the medium of human movement."

—William Morgan

*I*t was a hawk that ended my career. A great big, beautiful red tail that lofted, floated in the invisible updraft at the edge of a stand of tall eucalyptus. She hung in the sky like a painted kite on a string.

I ran by her, nearly as fast as my aging legs could carry me, slowed to have a look, slowed more to have a better look...and then stopped, gazing, wondering. Damn, she was a pretty bird.

Her head moved, body following, sharp eyes hunting the edge of the stand. I saw the hooked curve of her beak and watched her free-fall to a height of no more than forty feet, close enough that I imagined she was watching me, even wondering why I had stopped when all the others in front of me had kept moving down the wide, muddy trail much faster than I, while she scanned the soft earth for breakfast. That was the precise moment when I knew it was over.

Most people remember life-altering occurrences clearly. They can name the exact time and place, the activity in which they were involved, their companions, if any, and sometimes their exact feelings before *and* after the event. President Kennedy's assassination, the moment you proposed or were proposed to, a parent's death—snapshot memories in Technicolor, soundtrack included, that shape our lives from that instant until we ourselves pass away.

I never thought I'd have one of those to signify the end of my career as a professional athlete. No, I figured I'd just slowly burn out,
an ancient star losing its bright luster as it fell from the sky. I had
never planned a ceremonial farewell event or a send-off tour, replete
with opportunities to say goodbye to all those people and places
that had defined nearly half of my life. There would never be *that
moment.*

But there it was. She was. I was, just standing on the edge of a trail
watching a bird float in the shallow treetops, hunting for breakfast
while I subconsciously hunted for another life. Nothing out of the ordinary, really, except I was *supposed* to be running hard and fast. That's
what I had always done. That's what one does in a race. But I wasn't
racing; I was watching, bird-watching, for Christ's sake, an activity
appropriately associated with the older, more sedate crowd. An endurance sport it is not.

The hawk banked and trimmed, an eye on the horizon, an eye out
for small game, and maybe, just maybe, an eye on me.

The sound of foot strikes came up the trail, heavy breathing,
grunting almost. The rhythmic wisp of nylon shorts rubbing together,
shoes lifting, landing, lifting, landing—always forward toward an un-
seen but palpable goal: a PR, a top-ten finish, respect, money, a few
pounds shed, bragging rights around the water cooler. Whether the
goal was shallow or noble, the other guys I raced against (and now,
with my declining performance, the other women) always had a goal,
if not a raison d'être, for making themselves hurt the way they did. I
had lost my reason. I was watching a fucking bird fly. Just like that.

The first to pass me said nothing, silently gloating probably. "I
passed Tinley," he'd brag to his buddies after the race. The next one
slowed, but only in passing, and offered some homogenous form of
"keep it going." He had his job to do. And I had mine.

I returned to the task at hand and refocused my intent on moving toward the finish. I began a slow trot and then accelerated rapidly to something nearly definable as running. Just then I came upon
another runner, an age-group competitor who had started earlier in
the day and who should have been finished long ago. I passed him

carefully on the left on a narrowing section of trail now hidden inside a wide band of trees. I had nothing of real empathy to offer, so I said nothing at all.

Then it came. "Did you see the way her tail feathers spread out, like a peacock maybe, just before she rode the thermals towards the heavens?"

No, I didn't take any medals home that day. But later, when I climbed the steps to the plane that would carry me home, tired, sore, more than a bit confused, I carried with me a growing resolution to understand not so much what my life had been for the last twenty years, but what it would be for the next twenty, should I live that long. And what role physical movement would play through it all.

Would I find meaning and purpose in movement again? Would I dare to challenge others and myself in a race to prove something, *anything*? Or would I be content to stand off to the sidelines and ponder the aesthetics of flight, subconsciously looking for and living through this creature's movement?

I knew there were future challenges for me—intellectual, cerebral, existential. Probably lots of them. They just weren't staring me in the face at that moment. I was an athlete, dammit. I was a shark who would drown if he stopped swimming. But mostly I was lost and confused, a kid trying to find his way home.

I finished that race, skipped the massage tent, grabbed a towel, and headed for the beer stand. No one wanted to interview me. Fine. I had nothing to say that could be said in less than two hours and seven or eight beers.

I was feeing a lot of things, mostly sorrow. Sorrow for what I would never have again, sorrow for all the stupid shit I had done, and sorrow for the people out there who would run right by that hawk, obsessed and compelled toward a momentary finish line, a false Babylon of galvanized scaffolding, sponsors' banners, and the fleeting illusion that crossing that gate had tangible benefits. Where that feeling of sadness and clairvoyance came from, I'll never know. Maybe I had so much sorrow for myself that it was leaking out and projecting onto the others. I wouldn't call it pity, just raw, soul-wrenching angst.

Guilt started to creep in; guilt about not being at a son's soccer game or a daughter's cheerleading competition. And guilt is a powerful emotion, often disguising deeper feelings of remorse, confusion, and loss.

I needed a coping mechanism, another beer, a friend, a pen and paper to write it all down. Instead I went for a run, legs screaming, beer sloshing, eyes watering behind the sunglasses, wanting to hurt myself so I wouldn't feel the pain, a shark circling the ocean floor, knowing if the water should fail to pass through his gills, he dies.

You never learn anything when you're on top. You are in control, people have to listen to you, and so you talk, sometimes too much. All your time and energy is spent working out how to hang on to your throne and your kingdom, which by now you have convinced yourself rightfully belongs to you.

And you know what? It does. To get to the top of the heap, you have to pay your dues, develop your talent, kiss the right asses, say the right things to the media...and you have to do the work. More work than you ever thought possible. But it must end.

I ran into the great NFL quarterback Steve Young at a celebrity event on one of the first autumn Sundays in twenty years that he was not committed to playing football.

"How are you feeling Steve?"

"Weird," he said. "Definitely out of place."

If Steve Young had felt out of place, I was exactly where I needed to be—in the vortex, in a state of turmoil that might eventually lead to a process of healing. My life had been orderly, complete, as clear and purposeful as one who hates regularity could hope for. The clarity of sport had allowed the rest of me to be wild. It had been a hell of a lot of fun.

Now all that was gone, I assumed. Everything I had worked so hard for was slipping through my fingers, hour-glassed days I would never pull back. Things were about to change. I was going back to the real world and I was afraid, not of the work but of what I perceived as normalcy. My father died when I was fifteen, and I moved away to go to school a few years later. Since then I had never lived a normal life. I despised tedium and constant, humdrum and so-so.

The irony was that even though movement and change had defined me, this new challenge of self-exploration seemed far reaching, even daunting. That's when I began the conversations.

It might have been a form of prayer, or a kind of self-talk left over from my days of practicing sport psychology; it could have been harmless babble or profound discussion with an angel. These conversations or ruminations came without warning and didn't always yield answers. But they always made me ask the right questions.

It took me years to learn how to decode the messages, but eventually I could read the signs as if they were being delivered over my FM radio station, piped right into my brain. When you take a distant signal, filter it through the deepest part of your soul, and then send it back out, the answers can come back so crisp and simple and crystallized that you can't help but believe there is a greater power hiding in the confessional of clouds. But that's a long journey, and it can take many years.

She was beautiful wasn't she, hotshot? A real once-in-a-lifetime deal. I was out running back on the course, looking for my bird and my past.

"Well, yeah, that was a nice-looking bird but I've seen them before."

Years later, when my signal returned, I knew that answer was the beginning of my denial. I had seen hundred of hawks, but not this one, not now, not in this place and time.

I would hear from this voice again. No doubt. And it both scared and thrilled me.

Chasing a Dream

"The dream was always running ahead of me. To catch up, to live for a moment in unison with it, that was the miracle."

—Anais Nin

Every child has a hero. Heroes are important, and have been for eons. As a child, I only had one real hero. Even that turned out to be too many. He was my dad. When dads are good heroes to young sons, the mark is deep, indelible and irreversible. Superman, Zeus, Willie Mays, and John Wayne didn't make the cut.

My singular problem with having such a hero was that my dad died when I was fifteen years old, several years before I could have effectively evolved out of his image, and too soon to discover his fallibility, as we all must in our parents. I was stuck not only with an image of my dad as The Great Provider of All Things, but also with the gut-wrenching memory of watching him die slowly and painfully under the ravaging onslaught of cancer. One day he was thirty-eight, tan and fit, with a house full of kids and a life's worth of devoted friends. A year and a half later, weighing 130 pounds, with sunken, jaundiced eyes reaching out to some God with whom he may have made peace, he called each of his seven kids to his bed and said goodbye, be good, take care of mom. Like he was sending us off to camp.

He had fought the good fight, losing in the end to an indiscriminate and deadly enemy. My hero was gone and he would never be replaced. In later years, I admired the quiet mystique of Larry Bird and the never-say-die attitude of Steve Prefontaine, but they weren't Terry Tinley. And I suffered from this loss in ways that I am just now beginning to understand. I was left in that netherworld between child and adult where a teen begins to create his or her own true sense of self, moving back and forth between personal independence and the security of the parents. When my hero left me, I had not yet become an individual. I was stuck in a purgatory, sometimes a rebel without a cause, sometimes a child desperately lonely and in need of affection.

In one way, the experience made a mess of my life, then and now. And in another it set in motion a slow but constant march toward an understanding and framework of life that would not only validate my existence as a human being, but would eventually put me atop my own Hero's Pedestal.

I find the irony palpable at times. My father's death gave me the strength and independence to do things I never would have done had he lived. If he were alive today, I wonder if I would have been as good an athlete as I was. I *know* I would not have had as much difficulty as I did when Scott Tinley, the Athlete himself, died.

As a twenty-four-year-old paramedic, I could roll up on a multi-car traffic accident with several fatalities and direct cops and fireman like a hardened general, never once flinching or batting an emotional eye. I did my job with a precision beyond my years, never knowing where that skill came from. But even now, more than thirty years after his death, thinking and talking about my dad can break me down like a five-year-old with a skinned knee.

Sport was the guiding light that led me out of the netherworld where my father's death had left me. As a child I was never a great athlete. I had dwelled in the also-ran ranks of junior varsity and second string ever since the Maverick Little League Pee-Wee Bears "drafted" me as an eight-year-old walk-on. Junior high flag football, freshman basketball, sophomore baseball—it mattered little, I was average at best. And that somehow didn't fit well with my efforts to impress my hero. Dad of course only wanted me to do my best and be happy. But hell, I didn't know that. I had six brothers and sisters and I wanted to stand out. The wounds were deep each time I missed a shot or sat the bench.

There are moments in all of our lives that are so intensely emotional that if we lived to be a hundred years old, we could still pull them up from the recesses of our minds and replay them as if they happened only yesterday. My first game with the Pee-Wee Bears was such a moment. Sitting in the dugout, mitt in hand, I was ready to go out and play anywhere, to do anything, but the call never came. The coach, an old curmudgeon even then, is most likely dead by now. It would be easy for me to blindside him, but actually I should thank him.

He never put me in: He never let me play a single inning, even in right field, the Siberia of Little League. I was the only one who rode the pine for the entire six innings. When the game was over, I told my dad I wanted to hang around, maybe get a snow cone; he should go on without me. But he knew. Good parents always do.

And after I made the long, solitary walk home that night, making sure to steer clear of anybody I knew or didn't know, crying like the little boy I was, the damp night air fogging my breath, I arrived home a different person. I didn't know it then, but I know it now, as well as I know my own son.

I loved sports and everything I knew about the different games, even at that age. I wanted to play but, even more, I needed to. Coach Wills had denied me that chance. He had done more than embarrass me; he had taken away from me something that I didn't even know I needed—a chance to move, to be thrilled, to be needed.

I'm sure it was simple oversight on his part but years later, as one team sport after another came and went, I always remembered that first bad seed. I would be my own sportsman, and if I ever found the right sport, a damned good one.

> "When I was little, I remember realizing that every time I took the field, I did something good."
> —Boston Red Sox outfielder Johnny Damon

Six months before my dad checked out, the same day I was cut from the sophomore baseball team, I wandered over to the track.

Somewhere between discouraged and desperate, I asked with what innocence I could gather if I could join the track and field team. Of course, the coach snickered, just jump in with that group and follow them around the track until you barf.

To everyone's surprise, including my own, I not only held my lunch down but matched the team's best, stride for stride, during a speed workout of five one-mile repeats. I had found something I could be proud of. Something that my parents could come and see and then go home and brag to the neighbors about.

In the moldy-floored locker room, legs quivering with pain, standing lightheaded in the showers with my brethren, all was right with the world. My dad was too sick to watch me race that season, though. And by the time I had become the best distance runner at the school, he was gone. That cut was deep, but the blood would take time to spill.

At fifteen I was finally good at something. I could bury my troubles on the dirt straightaway, leave the pain and despair in the rutted curve, and forget that my dad was dying as I crossed the finish line first. The victories were hollow but they were something to grasp onto as I struggled to find meaning and stability. It doesn't seem like much now, but running was the only thing that belonged to me; they couldn't take it away from me like they had my hero. And so I ran. And when I got tired, I stopped, rested, and ran some more. I didn't realize it then, but I was running both toward and away from my past.

Back then, sports allowed me to feel something, what pro football Hall of Famer Joe Greene called "the environment." "People who are in sports," Greene said, "can walk out on to the field and just feel it, before anything is ever done...feel the environment."

For many athletes, that is how it begins: You "feel" something. Forget all the talk about destiny and natural talent and scholarships and three-year-olds with tennis rackets. More times than not, it begins innocently enough, with a gut feeling, a joy, a simple thrill.

Five years after my dad passed away, three years after high school graduation, thousands of miles later, I was still running. It was 1977 and I was a twenty-one-year-old college student working as a sailing instructor and living in an area of San Diego famous for its beaches, bays, and healthy population. Running had now taken on a different meaning, as it would more than once throughout my life. In 1977 it was a nice break from coursework, a way to burn off a morning hangover. I was still pretty good, mostly by accident, but not great; on a good day I could sneak into the top ten in a local road race. Competition at that level held only a passing interest for me. I would never be world class, and running by itself had become more of a way to relax. It was a diversion from the stress of earning enough money to pay the rent. It was fun.

I ran forty to fifty miles each week, mostly at an easy pace, sometimes with a bit more effort. I was okay with that. Additionally, I had begun to swim more, mostly because I had added another part-time job as a lifeguard. And because I didn't own a dependable car, I began commuting by bicycle, which rounded out my accidental cross-training regime.

All this changed in August of 1977 when I entered my first triathlon on Mission Bay's Fiesta Island. It was a casual affair, fewer than fifty competitors gathering on a Wednesday afternoon for a race listed as a "miscellaneous event" by the San Diego Track Club. I had watched one of these swim-bike-run affairs the previous summer and had been intrigued enough to inquire about the next event. "We only put on one or two of these things each year," the race director told me. "Keep an eye on the bulletin board next June."

Next June rolled around and I found myself competing in an event that included a four-mile run, an eight-mile bike ride, and a series of short swims and runs in and around the bay and this dirt spit of land with the ambitious name of Fiesta Island.

Think back to your first day on a new job where you ended up working for many years, or the first date with your future husband or wife. That is how I feel when I remember that first triathlon. At the time I didn't consciously attach any special meaning to the event, but over the years the memory has become richer and infinitely more intense. I can recall being nervous before the start for the first time since my high school league finals, a sure sign that I instinctively knew this race meant more to me than the casual 10Ks and half marathons that then made up my low-key competitive calendar. It wasn't the mixed-up order of events or even the surreal setting of the race, which began under a San Diego sunset. No, in my wizened look back, it could have only been the fact that triathlon embodied a devil-may-care, Southern California lifestyle that had defined my existence since the day my surfer parents brought me home from the hospital near the beach in a car with sand on the floorboards and a gym bag in the trunk. And it was the unique and eclectic combination of maverick personalities standing next to me on the starting line. They were regular, everyday folks—shopkeepers, accountants, salespeople. But they were shop-keepers who lived life on their own terms, accountants who knew how to have fun, and salespeople who knew that the trouble with normal is that it only gets worse.

I know now that I did not consciously choose this sport. Some things we get to choose, others choose us. That needs to be said twice.

I was beginning a lifespan, one of many bridges between the cradle and the grave. It was a new box of puzzle pieces all my own, a paint-by-number path with rewards along the way, and hardship, and something powerfully unknown and desirable at the end. This was a call that I could not ignore. There were never any guarantees, there never are. But I had no choice. Somehow I might have known that triathlon was a path out of that place where part of me was still stuck, a way for the boy to let his hero go by becoming someone else's. And now, as I suffer through the inevitable withdrawal from the sport that I ultimately and admittedly overidentified with, that statement is both a testimony to and an indictment of its powerful draw.

Indeed, not only was this new sport attractive enough for me to begin training for the next triathlon, should it ever happen, but I also subconsciously embraced the entire as-yet unformed concept of mul-tisport training and competition. I can remember coming home from that very first swim-bike-run affair, a third-place trophy in hand, and telling my roommate I had finally found "my sport."

I had one small problem, though. This new passion of mine was a narrow and underground "cult sport," comprising no more than a dozen races in the known world—kind of like falling in love with a girl and then finding out that she's married, gay, and lives in Katmandu. Still, I was unconcerned. She may have come to the party late and didn't have a lot to talk about, but she was there and I planned on making the best of our time together.

Climbing

"Between the idea and reality lies the shadow."
　　　　　　　　　　　　　　　　　　—T.S. Eliot

"That which makes you stronger can kill you in the end."
　　　　　　　　　　　　　　　　　—Scott Tinley, 2003

I am an athlete; I always have been. The definition will morph as my body grows older and my waistline enters a full-scale war with gravity. Whereas I once might have shuddered at the thought of finishing out of the top three at a major event, I may reach the point, if I'm lucky enough to live that long, where I would be equally troubled with a 5K time on the wrong side of thirty minutes. Regardless of what criteria I use to define myself as an athlete, the identity itself will never leave me. That much I know to be true.

By making that claim, I am affirming not so much a profession or an ideology, or even—to use an overused term—a *lifestyle*, but an encapsulating self-portrait. It will fade with time as all photographs do, and I may have it touched up with the latest technology, I may train harder for an event or two, but it will always stand sentinel to a portion of who I am.

It's odd, even frightening, for me to read these confessional and committed words. I mean, it's not like standing up and lamenting the loss of my job as an astrophysicist or as the CEO of a Fortune 500 company (people I definitely am not, as much as I admire their skills). Millions of people around the world can claim the title "athlete," each with his or her own rhyme and reason.

Why then do I squirm in my chair when I say that my athleticism—because it was a profession *and* a lifestyle and the core of my existence for most of my life—will help define me as long as I walk this earth? What is it in my admission that I played a boy's game for men's compensation that creates an emotional response in me that is unpleasant at best and downright scary at times?

It is this: A schedule had been arranged for my education, my return from the journey that I had taken in pursuing sport at the highest level. The game was over. And the work had begun. It was the cold, hard slap of fear that I would never again reach the dizzying heights of athletic success; that life in my mid-forties would become mundane, homogenous, watered-down; that I would never again stand atop the podium and watch people stand and clap for what I did, for who they thought I was, for what they wanted me to be? I was afraid that there would be a crisis of meaning in my life. But what is that fear, I thought? I still had my health, my family and friends, other athletic interests. If I really missed the competition, as many athletes do, I could find a new arena in which to compete. But it scared me that I went too far. Yes—I probably went way too far. And the fear was emanating from the unknown, as it often does.

While I didn't know it for sure, I was beginning to believe that I had gone "too far" by competing well past my prime, by over-identifying as an athlete, by letting other important aspects of my life slip away into some little crack that would not be so hard to extricate them from.

And while I thought it would be easy to leave sport, it would take deep study and thought before I was through with my "return," I would know more about athletic retirement than just about any academic or sports psychologist around. I would research it, write about it, and talk to hundreds of men and women in my position; and I would live it. I made sure there would be no unknown. If I was feeling a certain way about my retirement, I'd know why.

The journalist Bill Lyons once said that the lifelong professional athlete is the only member of our society who has to die twice. Others might contest that claim: the soldier returning from war, the career homemaker watching her last child leave the house for good, the twenty-nine-year-old dot.com millionaire who has reached his life's goals before his thirtieth birthday.

Some years ago, at the peak of my own game, I could not comprehend such a thought. Now, after having felt so fully the death of my other "self," the one who competed in nearly five hundred triathlons during a twenty-five-year career, I can say that I accept the sense if not the exact truth of the statement. I believe that a part of Scott Tinley the athlete has died, and another part can never be killed.

How is it that a society that devotes an entire section of the daily newspaper to sports coverage, a society that reveres the players of these games more than Nobel Prize-winning scientists, college professors, captains of industry, and politicians, can't figure out a way to deal with athletes once their time as players has ended? Could it be as simple as the idea that seeing "The Greats" aging reminds us that our own youth is passing too quickly?

I guess I shouldn't be surprised when people say, "Why should I be concerned about Joe Montana after football? He has enough money to do whatever he wants!" Or, "What difference does it make whether Pete Rose is ever allowed back in baseball? He's a fading memory of a lot of base hits and a little bit of gambling."

The athletic memories we hold dear tend to reflect our own youthful dreams and aspirations. If we think of Muhammad Ali, and thoughts of our own virile youth come to mind, all is well. But what if an image of Ali in recent years fills the mental picture screen? Silent, shaking, sorrowfully vulnerable in his battle against Parkinson's disease, well, there's a thought that is rapidly repressed and replaced with a memory of the younger, unconquerable fighter. If "The Greatest" can fall victim to a debilitating disease without a cure, what about the rest of us everyday folk? Are we next? And what of Christopher Reeves? If Superman is vulnerable, how are we to do battle with an enemy that attacks without reason or warning? It seems we only desire our Super-Jock Heroes when they can do what they are supposed to do: make us feel good. When they fail, we find someone else who can. Why should we care how athletes spend the rest of their days, whether they're playing golf or struggling with a painful addiction to drugs and alcohol? For much of the American public, it's irrelevant. These guys made their beds, let them lie in them.

The truth is, the fans are never so close to the former star as when they watch him fail at moves that were natural, even mindlessly easy, in his prime. The fan might say out loud, "Move on man, let somebody else have a turn," but inside, if the fan is honest with himself, he won't pity the fading star simply because he can't do it anymore. If the fan had the same courage as the aging athlete, he'd know that the connection comes in accepting that he too will grow old and fail.

> *"Do you have any idea what it's like? To run out through those concrete archways onto the crisp, green playing fields to the sound of 60,000 screaming fans? And to do it every Sunday for half the year?"*
> —Jerry Sherk, Cleveland Browns linebacker

Most of us dream of what it would be like to hit a baseball out of a ballpark, or cross the finish line of a marathon in first place. We let our minds carry us over the goal line, into the winner's circle, and up onto the podium. But how would it be to follow that career down, as all must go? How does it feel to live half your life in a bubble of athletic insulation, a privileged sacristy where the only requirement for salvation is to win? And then one day, all that is gone: the money, the fame, and the victories, all seemingly pointless because you have lost the most elemental requirement for existence—your sense of self.

Three-time Tour de France winner and one of America's greatest cyclists, Greg LeMond once told me that he wondered if maybe his life would have been better if he had just followed a simple, traditional path, like becoming a motorcycle mechanic.

This thinking, of course, is completely foreign to those who strive for all that a champion of LeMond's caliber stands for. How can he say that, they ask? Is he nuts? He's rich, he's famous, and he has accomplished more than most people ever dream of. Why would he want to work on carburetors instead?

Dreams are what drive us. As one Native American elder said, dreams are smarter than men. Even now, when my days of putting on the scarf, downing the sake, and jumping in the cockpit are over, I have dreams of success. But they do not involve crowded stands and sweaty bodies and earning more money in a day than I do in a year now. And Greg LeMond also has new dreams, ones that may ultimately be more fulfilling than winning one of the most difficult athletic contests on earth. LeMond was talking about the crisis and challenge in change, that fear of what Freud referred to as "turning neurotic misery into common unhappiness." Because once you have succeeded as Greg LeMond has, common unhappiness is entirely unacceptable.

Still we keep dreaming.

Why is this exit from sport so hard for top athletes? Why did I spend two years in a haze of confusion about who I was? Why is this transition different from a divorce, or the loss of a job, or the loss of a loved one? Life is full of change.

The answer is not simple. Each individual has his or her own ability to change, and a certain relationship to sport. For some, professional sport is just a temporary side trip before embarking on a *real* career. For others it is a way out of the financial hardship of inner-city life. And for many it starts out as a great way to have fun doing what they enjoy. Over the years, though, sport becomes far more than that. It becomes their family, their friends, their lover, their home, and their vessel for emotional growth; in short, it becomes their identity. Retirement robs them of a reason for getting up in the morning, of their dreams, their plans, their daily routine. Take it away and you rob them of their existence.

One study conducted by two sport psychologists found that 12% of the retired professional athletes polled stated that it took them six years to adapt to their new situation, while another 23% said it was a full two years before they felt totally adapted. During the course of my own study, I asked my friend Linda Buchanan, the top female triathlete in the world during the early to mid 1980s, how long it took until she felt "normal" again after retiring. Ten years, she said, ten years.

"To me," she recalled, "that was when new things in my life had preempted my involvement in triathlons. Nowadays, I can barely remember that I competed. I know it was me because I have the memories, but it was another lifetime." During that period Linda was successful in academia, business, and her personal life. The irony is that after being the best, you must redefine "normal," not just return to it, because after you've been somewhere very special for a very long time, everything is forever different.

Say you take ten years to reach your athletic peak, and then play for seven to ten years, and then use up another five readjusting to a normal existence. Well, you've eaten up a hell of a lot of your life. It had better be worth it, don't you think?

How does this happen anyway? When men and women decide to pursue a career in sport, to strive for athletic greatness, when they are willing to pay that lofty price, they must retain that identity long after their playing days are over. Complicating the problem, the public doesn't always know what to do with the old soldiered jocks. The jocks let it happen. And the fans encouraged it. They fed it, nourished it, and made it grow because they were raised on heroes. Heroes were in the bedtime books our parents read to us. They were on the posters we hung on the wall as teenagers. They were the ones our coaches told us to watch and emulate. And they are the ones that we live through vicariously in adult life, when our routine becomes too much to take. Our society has a place for heroes. But it has no place for ex-heroes.

Bringing them in to shake a few hands at a company meeting may be worse than ignoring them altogether. The message sent is that they are only valuable to us in their former lives. What about their new lives? Can we accept them as regular people, outside the spotlight of athletic entertainment?

After I stopped competing professionally, I went back to San Diego State University to finish a master's degree, the exact place I had left to turn pro almost twenty years earlier. It was the only substantial task that I had quit in my life. I used to have bad dreams about it: I would wake up the night before big events in a cold sweat, not having dreamt of losing the race but of missing classes or getting failing grades. I took that as a sign, and after I retired I told my wife Virginia that I'd find a paying job soon and she went back to work. We cut back on our expenses and off to school I went, empty pages in my notebooks and in my head. I was prepared for the challenge, but my wife wasn't as excited.

"S. T.," she'd say, "you worked so hard to make a name for yourself in sport. You could coach or do television commentary, or make triathlon videos. Why make it so hard on yourself? Why start all over again?" My kids, thirteen and nine at the time, had grown up with Dad the Jock. If they had expected me finally to be like the other dads and climb into a suit and tie, to join the fray of regularity, they never let on. I think they were secretly proud that I marched to a different tune, that I was home during the day, that I had worn shorts to every job I ever held, that I played handball with them at lunch.

But how could I tell Virginia that the professional sportsman part of me was gone, dead, left the building with Elvis? I wanted to write, teach at the highest level, learn, and exercise my mind in the same way I had my body—with a sense of passion and commitment. How could I tell her it might be seven to ten years before I would earn a third of what I was making at my peak in triathlon? I wanted to be honest. I also knew that the divorce rate for retired athletes in the major professional leagues was 60% to 70% post-retirement. Sadly, it made sense. You become a new person, one often quite different from the one your spouse married. I wouldn't have blamed Virginia if she had walked out during that dark period when I struggled for identity. Still, I knew that my only chance at finding happiness again was to follow my instincts and my knowledge of who and what I was. At that point the athlete in me had gone dormant, and the creative, introspective bohemian had woken up.

After two weeks in school, it was obvious that I was better off hiding my past athletic success. I wanted to be judged as a student, not an ex-jock looking to dabble in something new to fill his time. When people found out about my past, my future was on trial, or at least that's how I perceived it. Soon my obsessive nature took hold and my original program of study seemed stale and unimaginative. I had to create an interdisciplinary Masters in Social Psychology of Sport and then

apply to enter the elite MFA program in creative writing simultaneously. I was doing three or four Ironman events a year all over again. I
wanted knowledge, and I wanted it now, dammit. As one of my friends
said, all I had done was "trade Nikes for Nietzsche." Writing papers,
doing research, teaching lower division classes, grading papers—all of
this made my old forty-hour-a-week training programs seem easy.

One night during a short break from a three-hour seminar, a class-
mate probably half my age, who was dressed in black and had too
many pierced body parts to count, offered me a cigarette, flicking the
pack to make only one cigarette phallically emerge, as only smokers
can. I stared at the smoke and then at him for a moment too long.

"What's wrong? Don't smoke this brand?"

"No, I'm sorry. It's just that…I don't think anybody has ever offered me a cigarette before in my entire life."

He took half a step back, looked at me queerly, and asked if I had
been living in a cave.

Sort of, I told him. Sort of.

Where is the success in all of this? Where is the feel-good part that
draws a tear from your eye? Where are the stories of those who made
a smooth, seamless transition back into the Real World? Oh, for sure,
they exist. But we don't hear about them. Is it noteworthy that a former pitcher from the Los Angeles Dodgers is doing color commentary
and owns an interest in a Ford dealership?

Similarly, we rarely hear about the ones who struggled, who hit
bottom, who went broke, went to jail, tried suicide. I know a number
of ex-pros who went on to become successful, well-adjusted business
men and women. Most of them have a happy family life, kids, money
in the bank—all the pugmarks of achievement as defined by our society. They seem happy.

And I have met those who sit on the porch all day, bottle in hand,
too poor to even spend the night, always talking about the good old
days. They count a time that has forgotten them. Stuck.

They might exist in barstool legends, but they aren't sure who
they are because everybody else thinks they know. And when they
dream, it's almost always in reverse.

No Compromise

"I am afraid of many things, most of which have already happened or will fail to occur."
—From the author's journal, August 3, 2001

*H*enry David Thoreau once wrote, "The mass of men lead lives of quiet desperation." As a young man, hungry for achievement, willing to bet the farm, I could not understand that. Why would anyone settle for less than the best? Life was to be lived on the edge. Idealism was king, compromise was for losers.

I knew I had "the right stuff." How I knew, I am not sure. I guess some of it was confidence earned through early results. Some of it was an innate knowledge of my ability to persevere when others gave up. And some of it was simply a good old-fashioned hunch.

The first race of any stature that I won—my first victory that was something other than a "club workout" and that had a real live awards ceremony with something like a free pair of shoes for the winner, or a coupon for a free steak dinner at a local restaurant—was called the Del Mar Days Triathlon. Ironically, the swim was off the same beaches where I still work as a lifeguard in the summer, the bike course sent cyclists near the house we have lived in for sixteen years, and the run followed trails over which I must have logged ten thousand miles since. It was a gray summer morning, "June gloom" we call it on the coast, and I felt very proud of my accomplishment. I also felt a shift in what competition meant to me. I had never thought of myself as overly competitive, maybe because of all the disappointment in my childhood sporting quests. This win though, and the feeling of instant self-esteem, awoke a long-dormant beast. After *this*, I knew I could win again. I had been given just a lick of the sweet drug and I would be asking for more.

How do athletes reach the point where they can cut all ties to normal, day-to-day life and focus all their time and energy on the sport? It is not a straightforward process. Everything must fall into place, the stars of possibility, fate, and circumstance all lying in perfect alignment, creating a window of opportunity which the athlete must not only recognize but be willing to jump through without hesitation. And though I didn't recognize it at the time, my stars were beginning to line up. One of them was plain old luck.

In 1980 I took a job as a paramedic, working a fireman's shift, twenty-four hours on, twenty-four hours off, with an occasional break of four or five days off in a row. I averaged about eleven full days and nights a month at the fire station, which allowed me gobs of time to train. And that is what I did. If luck is where preparation meets opportunity, I had both handed to me on a silver platter.

I was twenty-four years old with an unknown future and an unfinished master's degree, unable to commit to marrying Virginia, the woman who would become my wife, and grossly underpaid for this new job I had just spent a solid year training for. But I was young, healthy, in love, and working in a fire station with a bunch of crazy older guys who I could see growing up to be just like. Life was good.

Paramedic school had been the most difficult intellectual challenge of my life. I had lied about my experience to get one of the coveted new positions in the city of San Diego; when the notice of acceptance came for a job that I knew would change me deeply, I told Virginia and my younger brother Jeff, who were both living with me at the time, "I'm in for it now."

I knew I was smart enough to get through the extremely difficult training, but now I would have to apply myself. This would be the first real test of my ability to focus on one serious task, to get the job done. There was something else too. I sensed that I could make a difference; I could matter to people who were gravely sick and injured. I could poke fun at the death that had claimed my father, dance around its ugly edges. I could snatch people from its claws and tell death to fuck off—I'm on duty now. Growing up as one of seven kids, a marginal student, a marginal athlete, here was my first chance to do something of substance. My life would matter because it mattered to someone else.

Working as a paramedic had a profound effect on me. There were nights when the calls would keep coming—gunshot wound, stabbing, vehicle accident, man down—and I would step out of my own skin, like a snake molting, shedding my history and my future just to feel alive in the present. Seeing people so sick and debilitated gave me a true appreciation for the human body, for how resilient and fragile it could be. One second you could be an eighteen-year-old kid racing an eighty-horsepower "crotch rocket" motorcycle over to your girlfriend's house, a few beers in your head, a building lump in your pants, and then a block from your bliss you might miss a turn, wrap your lithe body around a light pole, and lie there knowing in your heart of hearts that you will never be the same young man again. Nope, not even close.

Sometimes we'd roll up on kids like these and go to work shoving IVs into them, pinching off spurting arteries with small instruments or fingers, going about our jobs as quickly and efficiently as we could, impassionate and stoic on the surface but inside knowing it could've been any one of us. In the more horrific accidents, the lucky ones were already dead.

Those didn't bother me as much as the ones we lost on the way to the hospital. I took that very personally, arrogantly in retrospect, as if I was the guy who decided who lives and dies. I'd become invested in the lives of the ones who I felt were *supposed* to live—the kids, the young girls who forgot to put on a seat belt, the older folks who had worked a lifetime dreaming of their golden retirement—all of them ripped from our care without any rhyme or reason that I could make out. And my only defense was a better offense: I got good at it. I knew my meds, I could read telemetry like a cardiac intern, I took control of trauma scenes like a grizzled old cop. One day I yelled at a couple of highway patrol officers for being too slow in getting the gurney out of the ambulance. To them I was a cocky kid who had embarrassed them in front of their peers. When I returned from the hospital to the fire station, they were there waiting for me.

"Hey buddy, cool it with the big mouth, huh?" one of them said.

I wasn't backing down. "You were affecting the patient care. That's part of your job chippie."

He was twice my age, twice my size, and I could tell he wanted to throw my punk ass against the wall so bad it hurt. I was in way over my head, but I couldn't figure out where my strength was coming from.

Later, when things quieted down, the captain asked to see me.

"Tinley, people die every day. You'll never last in this business if you care too much."

We didn't feel like heroes. It was a job that had to be done. But some years later, sometimes even now, in the ordinary hours of life, I feel good about what we did. Damn good.

I had been a party to something essential, something profound and unnamable. I heard what the captain was saying but still this elevated sense of existence had mixed with my own blood.

So I tried not to care and to carry out my job with skill and precision, and then I packed my shit in the morning and went home to work out. That's what I did on my days off—work out. Even though triathlons were few and far between back then, more an underground cult event than a bona fide sport, I had lots of time off, plenty of demons to exorcise, and a growing sense of confidence.

And so I trained, an hour a day at first, then two, then four, and then I carried it back to the job. I could usually convince my partner to find a centrally located park that I could run around, radio in hand, hoping that the sick and injured would leave me alone. I lifted weights at the station. When we came back from a stabbing, I'd do a hundred sit-ups; if we had a patient with chronic pulmonary disease, I'd carry a fire hose up and down the steps. My life had focused on the body. I was running all the time now, away from death and dying, toward a sport that was like a fountain of youth.

A life with physical fitness as its central theme is not for everyone. In fact, the vast majority would soon crumble due to physical injury, mental burnout, lack of motivation, or simple boredom. For me though, at that period in my life, it was perfect.

Triathlon offered me an opportunity to cut away all the emotional "fuzzies" in my life; it offered an immediate solution to the monumental task of finding my purpose in life. Helping the sick and injured, even the rush of an occasional big fire, was rewarding, but the work was taking a toll. Despite my best efforts to remain emotionally detached, it felt as if all the trauma I was exposed to was still leaking into my psyche. The filter I had erected wasn't doing its job. I tried working for another fire department, I thought about moving up the ladder to engineer or captain, but it was no use. The job had served its purpose, and much more of it would have been destructive. I had seen too much shit, too much pain and suffering. I was just a twenty-five-year-old beach rat trying to find his way in life, not Mother Theresa. I think now that, even as I tried to be distant, to act like the cool technician, I was afraid that this role might become real and I truly would lose the capacity to feel.

I walked into the chief's office and said I was done. He was smoking a pipe at the time and thought I was joking.

"No, really Chief. I don't want to be exposed to life's underside anymore."

"Okay, Tinley, how much time can you give me to replace you?"

"None," I told him. "I'm afraid I'll make a mistake."

"You just did kid. You just did."

I took away with me a feeling of having done something extraordinary. I had seen the shit, the parts of life that are not spoken of at the dinner table. And I knew that at any moment I could lose everything, even myself. But I doubted I would lose that feeling of making a difference, of having a kid look me in the eye and thank me for helping his mother.

Somehow, somewhere, I would find that feeling again, that intangible gift of doing exactly what you know in your heart you are supposed to do. I was beginning to understand how I would live.

▼ ▼ ▼

"I always wanted my life to revolve around the Sun in some mutual automaticity and sense of complementary color, like a cold beer at sunset or a gas station in the desert. Yeah, I had stars in my eyes, but I always knew that the Sun was more star than the stars themselves."
                    —From the author's journal, January 18, 1981

As an athlete grows into himself, creating or redefining his own identity, his sport becomes an integral part of his being. It happens slowly at first, but if he is going to make it to the top, it must happen. No one is immune. You may think you are making the decision—that by practicing long hours every day or by accepting a scholarship or by entering a major event that you are in control of your athletic life. But in the beginning it just happens. You feel a true love, an attraction so powerful that it cannot be ignored, although you may not understand its powerful grip until long after you have quit the game.

"You like going out there and throwing the ball up, and just seeing if it goes in," Kobe Bryant told *The Sporting News*. "That's basically what we do; we just make it more complicated."

Triathlon was still a small sport in the early 1980s, very uncomplicated. That suited me fine. I needed time to hone my craft before athletes with real talent began to take notice. Of course, after winning a few events, making the podium in a few more, I began to gain the self-confidence needed to compete at the highest levels. To win races of note you need a deep-seated belief that *you* are the best out there, that *you* deserve to win, that it is not so much your privilege as your right. This is no different from any other profession. I have a friend by the name of Jim Rice who is a cobbler. He owns a tiny shop where he regularly works ten to twelve hours a day replacing worn high heels and polishing expensive Italian leather. But what Jim lives for are the days when world-class athletes from various sports wander in on someone's recommendation and ask if he can tweak a cycling shoe cleat or lower the buckles on a moto-cross boot. And he does so with great care and precision. Everybody in the San Diego sports scene has heard of Jim Rice's Sole Performance because Rice knows that if he puts his creative time and energy into it, he can make any athlete the perfect shoe. One time I watched the cycling legend Greg LeMond walk into a party, ignore all the famous athletes and the media types, and go straight up to Jim Rice. "You're the shoe god, aren't you?" LeMond asked. For men and women like Jim Rice, belief in yourself is not an option. It is a requirement.

For me, it became a crusade. What I lacked in innate physical talent and skill, I made up for with a tenacious training regime and a supreme confidence. If I was logging more miles than my competitors, with a greater degree of intensity, I not only deserved to win—it was my destiny. So it is with world-class athletes: Their self-image is nearly godlike, as presumptuous as that might sound. If I had self-centered tendencies before, triathlon was the perfect vehicle for me to exercise that narcissism. As Jerry Sherk, a defensive back for the Cleveland Browns, once said, "We felt like gods but we knew we were pretenders."

Several things had to happen for me to center all my efforts on becoming the best. First, I needed a life structure that would not "distract" me from focusing all my time and effort on training and racing. This would not be easy.

In June of 1981, Virginia and I were married. Where I was frenetic and edgy, she was conservative and assured. Whereas my future was tumultuously uncertain, hers was secure and solid. Quite often we marry our opposites in an effort to complete some psychic circle. But I was very much in love, and she was supportive beyond reason.

In 1981 there was yet to be any prize money in the sport of triathlon. The only sponsorship I received after coming in third in the Ironman Triathlon World Championships was a free case of E.R.G. (Electrolyte Replacement with Glucose), the very first true "athletic drink," which was developed by Bill Gookin, a high school chemistry teacher and a friend of mine. The drink, which you could only get from Bill himself, had a small following within the San Diego Track Club. So I was now the proud owner of twenty-four twelve-ounce servings of what Bill affectionately called *GookinAid*. I was on my way. Somewhere.

In the previous twelve months I had gotten married, bought a house, and started a more "normal" job, coordinating instruction for the Mission Bay Aquatic Center. It was by no means a traditional occupation—I was teaching surfing, sailing, waterskiing, and paddling on the shores of San Diego's Mission Bay. But it required me to be there fifty hours a week, so I felt like I was being sucked into the hunt for the Great American Dream, an empty pursuit, I felt, and one that went against my rebellious nature.

My job was cool though, I had a great wife, a little cottage a few blocks from the beach, and some great friends to party and surf and train with. I had no right to complain about a thing.

A few weeks after I started the job, I convinced my sympathetic boss to let me go back to the Hawaiian Ironman one more time—"just to get this triathlon thing out of my system," my memo request stated.

That was a lie, however, and what happened redirected my attention back to the sport so fast that even I could not have predicted its overruling effect. I won the biggest triathlon in the world, beating the best there were in record time. And though I swore it wouldn't pump up my ego, in hindsight I now know that one cannot keep the drug of victory from seeping in.

The more introspective athletes know that. Al Leiter, the outstanding New York Mets pitcher, marveled at the effects of fame in an interview: "The other day I was walking with some friends in Manhattan and a kid walked by, he had a Mets shirt, [number] 22. I thought it was just a generic Mets shirt. I turned around, it had 'Leiter' on it. I just walked by and here he is wearing my jersey."

Former Philadelphia Phillies outfielder Doug Glanville told *The Sporting News* about hearing the crowds: "It's like you're on stage...Oh, I can't wait to hear that crowd."

But what is the meaning of this adoration? Is it a perk of a game played for near-mortal stakes? A perk of the job? A benefit that comes from having paid your dues through countless hours of practice?

And what of the athlete who abuses that benefit? Heaven knows there are many who find trouble easily, and thousands of fans who just can't believe that athletes might not be appreciative of the gifts they have been given. What? Twelve million dollars isn't enough? You need fourteen? And now you're using cocaine and getting into bar fights?

I felt the same way about crybaby pros. If I was headed for the ranks of professional sport, what would become of me?

These were the types of questions that ran through my mind after that first big awards ceremony in Hawaii. My brother Jeff had placed third and there was much to celebrate. We had trained together. We were blood brothers.

But there was deep confusion running through me along with the blood that had delivered the oxygen to my muscles only hours before. I knew I shouldn't get too used to this feeling. It would be addictive. This "vacation" had wiped out our savings, and I had to get home to work, to cut the lawn, to hold up the image of normalcy that I was desperately trying to run away from. It seemed to me very similar to when I was a paramedic. I wanted to care but I was afraid of the costs. Now, standing in front of a thousand people on their feet, clapping, there was some strange governor slowing my feelings. I should have felt happier; I should have been a more gracious champion.

I was this hero standing atop the podium. I heard my name called and the sound of the crowd as they offered their collective applause. In my head, I knew I had done something great and deserved recognition for the hard work invested. And in my heart I humbly accepted their acclaim, thanked those who had helped with the cause, and stepped down into emotional ambiguity. It could have been some sort of defense mechanism. It could have been that my dad wasn't there to see it. Maybe I felt that if I risked it all, I could lose it all. Hell, I didn't know.

But part of me remained atop that victory stand, unable to remove myself from my new home. That part couldn't be pried off easily and, sensing some value in leaving a bit of myself up there, I let that piece go into the hallowed hall. What I didn't realize is that given enough trips to that sacred place, there would be nothing left of myself to function in normal life, the life to which I must eventually, and traumatically, return. Perhaps I was afraid that my entire self would be left sitting on the dais, waiting for one more roar from the crowd.

When I went to the awards dinner and ceremony the night after the race with my wife, my brother, and my good friends and training partners Steve Perez and Brian Chadwell, the event was sold out. My friends tried to talk us past the rather large Samoans taking tickets at the door.

"Hey these dudes got first and third. Man, you got to let us all in." They weren't buying any of it. They didn't know Jeff or me. Why should they? The door was shut, the winners were surely inside, and we were posers. Virginia had mentioned that we should buy tickets in advance, but my victory had fueled my rebellious nature. Rules didn't apply to winners.

How is it that you won and couldn't get into the ceremony?

Some guy from Anheuser-Busch, the new title sponsor, came around and asked us if we would like to sample a case of this new beer they were launching, Budweiser Light. Well, we jumped on that, went around to the back of the building, sat on the curb, and sampled for awhile until we could hear the awards being given out through the open kitchen door. The last sixer went to the cooks who let us slip by and we were in.

"There is a truth I understand now," says George McGinnis, a retired forward who played with the Indiana Pacers. "When all is said and done, all I will be is the answer to a trivia question."

McGinnis's comment is harsh, but in many ways it rings true. How is it that I remember sneaking into that awards dinner more than I remember running the last mile of the race? Maybe it has to do with the fact that it was a shared experience as opposed to a powerful yet solitary one.

Athletes are lucky if they have close friends, friends who knew them before they made The Show. These friends will contribute to the athlete's humility. Sometimes it's a quiet talk, other times a reminder during a heated argument.

I was lucky in that respect. If I ever showed signs of an inflated ego—and I did on plenty of occasions, whether or not I realized it—I was gently but firmly brought back to earth with a, "Bro, you are *not* that cool."

Some athletes are better than others at putting up filters that let through just enough of the success, so that they can stand up, thank the crowd, accept their praise, and then move on. Very few are prepared for that situation. It's not something that you practice.

I was never good at that, and at times my resistance to praise was perceived as aloof and distant. Being a good champion is not easy. I might have been a rebel, but I wasn't a gambler. I had gambled before with emotions and lost. I could think of myself as a winner, a deserving victor, but the image of the graceful champion was elusive and frightening.

It would take me twenty years of self-exploration to solve this puzzle. By then, I was long past winning any big events. Dissecting it in print became my mode of expression.

When I returned from Hawaii that first year, the folks at the Mission Bay Aquatic Center threw me a little surprise party and, for effect, they invited the press. I remember feeling very uncomfortable, the hot lights blinding me, the camera in my face, the questions about how it felt, how did I train, what's next? I was still confused. Did this mean I was a pro athlete? Did one event with three hundred competitors that would air on ABC's *Wide World of Sports*—sandwiched between ice dancing and a NASCAR race—mean that I was on my way to fame and fortune? The TV show would get me a few calls from old friends, maybe a shoe sponsor. The koa wood trophy for first place did little to pay the rent that month. I had just conquered one of the greatest endurance contests in the world. And now I had to be at work on Monday morning, making sure that all the little sailboats were ready for class.

I was twenty-six and my future had not gained any post-college clarity; I had very little idea of what I wanted to be when I grew up, and it wasn't, as the "career indication" tests in high school had indicated, a fire watcher. Now, with a few months of serious training and one day's competition, my future was even less clear. I wasn't cut out to be a hero. But if it could keep me out of a suit and tie for a few years, heck, I'd give it a go.

My boss was Glen Brandenberg a bright and tenacious visionary. Glen was a real-life Peter Pan who once bet three of his coworkers a thousand dollars each that he would be the last to get married; he knew better. Glen never said anything at the time but he was watching, noting my gentle but unmistakable metamorphosis. To his credit, he never mentioned my expanding lunch hour as my noontime runs increased from four to six to eight to ten miles. He never mentioned that I left right after work to get in a bike ride before dark instead of heading to the local pub with the staff. I think he knew that what I had seen and felt in Hawaii was just the beginning. I had tasted that drug; I had heard the roar of the crowd. How could I come back and make sure all our sailboarding instructors weren't hungover the morning they were scheduled to teach a class?

But that is what I did. It was one of the ongoing lessons in humility that I would receive over the years. Glen told me I could always quit and follow my athletic dream if that was what I wanted.

"But G.B.," I replied, "this is one of the best jobs on the planet. How could I ever top it?" He rolled the ends of his mouth up, said nothing, and walked away.

The Myth of Sport and Sporting Warriors

"We are meant to outgrow ourselves, the only question is how gracefully and healthy we can do it."
—Anonymous

*W*hat if your dreams came true? What if you realized your little boy's dream of hitting a World Series grand slam? Or you achieved your little girl's fantasy of dipping your head so the president of the International Olympic Committee could drape the gold medal around your neck, the national anthem playing in the background, tears welling up in your eyes? What if they came true? What would it mean?

What if I saw Coach Wills, my old Little League coach, buying milk in a convenience store one spring afternoon. Would I walk up to him and ask if he remembered a skinny blonde kid in 1964, the bench warmer of the Bears, the bench warmer whose blood is on his hands? Or is it gold? Would I shake his hand and say hi? Or walk away in disgust?

No. I'd walk up to him and say, "Hello Coach Wills. I have a son now. I coach his teams. And everybody plays. Have a nice day."

But that is the talk of a retired athlete, one who has had his dreams fulfilled. And paid the price of living that dream.

Every athlete keeps certain memories—playing in that first game, or hitting that first home run—which are much more significant than ordinary memories of long-lost physical acts. An act that takes on an unfading significance, which stays with you long after countless other occurrences have been lost or repressed, becomes a myth. That is why my Pee-Wee Bears are mythic and why they will stay with me all of my days. The meaning is found in the story itself, the story that constantly re-energizes the feeling; it isn't urban legend or selective memory—it's real not only because it happened, but because the meaning attached to it gives it a mythic quality. And its purpose guides my life in ways that I am only now beginning to understand.

An athletic myth can be differentiated into sensory myth, commodified myth, and real myth. Sensory myth is what the fans see happening in front of them, what the athlete himself feels and experiences with all his senses during some significant event. The commodified myth is propagated by the media to elevate the story. Sports reporters have been mythologizing the sporting experience since before the beginnings of newspapers, radio, and television, since word of mouth could pass along the story with enough embellishment to make it larger than the event. A good story told around the town square would *sell* the storyteller to his audience. The mass media's purposeful manipulation of sport today is simply a grotesque exaggeration of that.

My mother has a framed front-page headline from my first Ironman victory hanging in her living room. It's from some local paper called the *Kona Today* or the *Hawaii Gazette*, something like that, where all of 2,500 people may have seen it that day in February of 1982. Under a photo of me crossing the finish line the caption reads, "Tinley Sets Ironman Record" in bold print.

Over the years, she has remodeled her living room half a dozen times but somehow, next to the changing original oils and scenic prints of mountains and rivers, the framed headline has stood sentinel in the same corner of the room, never fading, never hanging crooked. I mean to ask her about it every time I see it. After all, that was a lifetime ago. She has fifteen grandchildren. One of them must have gotten a small write-up in a local paper for *something*.

But I can't and I don't. The news clipping set inside an old brown-gold frame has become part of the myth, once commodified, now made real by the many conversations it must have prompted. I'm sure it means something to her, otherwise it would be in the back closet with a thousand other potential reminders of a family's success.

Real myth emerges when the meaning is taken from the myth, from the experience itself. When athletes are able to find enough meaning or lesson in their experiences, and that sensory connection stays with them, they can become a part of that myth, woven in time, the fluidity of memory hardening with time, becoming a form of raw truth to guide them should they allow it.

While my sensory connection to parts of my past may have faded, for others, it may still mean something. People often speak of an athlete's glory days in mythic language, reliving a memory of having "been there when he hit that ball clean out of the park." But truer myths are built through the unspoken word: the climber who puts up a new route and tells no one about it, the twenty-year-old photograph never moved from its rightful place.

One of my early writing professors is married to an ex-NBA player, an English teacher and poet by the name of Tom Meschery. I've spoken with him before but don't know him well, yet I've seen some of his poetry published in literary anthologies. I admire his work. One poem in particular is a tribute to the late Wilt Chamberlain and is quite good. Some years after first reading this poem I was told that he played with Wilt the night Chamberlain scored one hundred points. Meschery's poem took on mythic qualities for me because in our short conversations, he never mentioned anything of his own writing, his own NBA career, or his relationship to Chamberlain. In a sporting culture where "in your face" mentalities often prevail, an understated approach is refreshing and somehow reminds us of the nobler side of sport.

In many ways, the sporting hero assimilates the warrior myth. He or she has the warrior's heart, the need to be needed. The mantle of responsibility is thrust upon them and they must choose the life. Yes, modern day professional athletes are entertainers. They fulfill a need in the public, but at a very raw, essential level they have the opportunity to perform heroic-*looking* feats of physical capability, feats that become myth in the eyes of the fans, through the lens of the media. And meaning is found in the experience for the performer too. The question of whether or not they deserve the title of "warrior" has much to do with semantics, or the interpretation of the term in the context where it is presented.

There were no warriors in my recent bloodline, not the kind that fought and killed in wars. As far back as I could trace, not a single man or woman fought in a war for this or any other country. My grandfathers slipped between WWI and WWII, my father side-stepped the Korean War with a stint in the Coast Guard, and just as I was careening out of control into teenage rebelliousness, the Vietnam conflict looming ahead like a neighborhood bully lying in wait for a smartass kid, they halted the draft. For a hundred years or more, my immediate family was spared any killing field by the chance of birth date.

An uncle, on the other hand, spent twenty-two years flying jets in the Air Force. Three tours in Nam and to this day, he will not speak of Southeast Asia or UFOs. He was a sixth-generation Southern California native like the rest of siblings, raised on the beaches of Malibu. But war aged him faster than all of us, and even as I watch him fight the good fight of growing old, I see him not only as my mom's sister's husband, a tall lanky man who surfed with my dad, but also as a warrior who flew F-4s because that was his job. Regardless of the ethics and moralities behind the Vietnam War, his country told him he was needed and he went off to do what he was told, slowly, ignominiously, paying for that blind loyalty with a back operation here, an undiagnosed malady there, and decades of living many miles from any coast. My Uncle Bill defines the unique morphing of athlete and modern day warrior. His mind and his eyes are clear, his heart and his bones cloudy.

Perhaps sport's greatest gift to the world is in its substitute of defeat for battlefield death.

Part of the role of sport is to cheat death by creating the image of immortality. Whereas the soldier knows he can die at any moment, it is a struggle for the athlete and the public to have any concept of a hero in his prime ever becoming anything else. Most athletes themselves can confuse personal heroics, myth, and incredible athletic talent; for them to see themselves as old and weak makes it difficult to be young and strong. It is not an easy paradigm to unravel.

Indeed, we can easily confuse our heroes. Most athletes never go beyond donating a few hours to a charity, lending their name to a foundation, signing autographs. For some, it's not so much that they aren't willing, they just don't understand. Nobody is taught how to be a hero or a living myth. There are no role model schools. And for others, the ones who abuse their privileges, as well as their coaches, friends, spouses, fans, and most of all themselves, the problem is much deeper. It is unfair if not myopic to make blanket statements about prima donnas who can't seem to stay out of trouble. Their problems are often complex and deep-seated. Still, the fans who pay the ticket price and only want to be entertained, to see a good game, well, they too have a voice. Sometimes those who need each other the most are the furthest apart.

The scholar Joseph Campbell was once asked if most leaders and heroes live close to the edge of neuroticism. He replied that yes, some do, that it is part of their "genius" that has been bestowed upon them. One immediately thinks of the burden of artistic gift, that the most talented artists look at the world in a different way, a way that ostracizes them. Van Gogh's ear, Michael Jackson's eerie and oft-changing appearance, Beethoven's inner demons—that sort of thing. Truly gifted athletes are no different.

Heroes don't necessarily have to glide like Michael Jordan or swing a club like Tiger Woods. They simply have to do extraordinary things, selflessly, in the service of others. In the traditional definition of a hero, physical talent has nothing to do with the label.

I have known many professional athletes in my years. Some recognize just how lucky they are. They do what they can to give back, partly because they want to, partly because they need to. Others sense that a little public charity is advisable in maintaining the benefits of athletic celebrity. And there are still those who refuse the entire frame, trying to live their athletic and non-athletic lives as if they were one and the same, pretending they are not famous and rich and a sought-after commodity due to their talent and exposure.

It is difficult to say if one group is happier than another. You can only look at individual cases and form your own opinion. The question of whether one's life has meant anything does not often come up at the dinner table. It is usually reserved for the final days, when we balance our karmic accounts.

"I am not obsessed by the question of whether or not people would know my name a hundred years from now," wrote tennis great Arthur Ashe in his memoir, *Days of Grace*. "But I did want to achieve something more than I had accomplished on the tennis court."

In the last five years of his life, Ashe devoted his brilliance and strength to many worthy causes, including the fight against racial prejudice, the battle against AIDS, and the active opposition to South African apartheid. It is safe to say that Arthur Ashe accepted fully the responsibility of the mythic hero; he interpreted his experiences and gifts on the tennis court and returned to give back, to complete the "hero's journey" that Joseph Campbell has written about. It is the journey that begins when the hero is chosen by fate, accepts his or her challenge, and if successful, returns to the "tribe" or the rank and file of the *everyman* to tell us what they've learned in their quest.

In modern day application of this legend, Ashe's journey was complete. By any definition, he was a hero.

Five-time Olympic gold medalist Eric Heiden is no different. After winning all those medals at the 1980 Olympics, the speed skater declined numerous endorsement opportunities and returned to finish his undergraduate work at Stanford before applying to medical school. Can you imagine turning down a chance to be on a Wheaties box because you had a biology final to study for? Years later, Heiden is a successful orthopedic surgeon. He has built another life after sport, a life based on healing people, not doing ads for ACME widgets.

I've known Heiden for many years and have watched him go from speed skating to cycling to medical school to fixing broken bones and torn rotator cuffs. To me what is mythic about Eric is the seamlessness of his transitions between professions, between lives.

"I have had a life after sports," he told me. "A lot of people end up really living in the past. It's one of those things, the older you get the better you were! It just gets worse and worse."

"How so?"

"If people ask me about...what is my greatest accomplishment, I could say I was a speed skater, but in the grand scheme of things, does it mean all that much that I can skate four hundred feet of track faster than anybody else? What I do now is much more meaningful."

And possibly more mythic.

Change in the Air

"There will come a day when some of these fellows draw that pension money years from now and they will probably have completely forgotten how they earned it. They got it because a lot of guys stuck out their necks."

— Tim McCarver, professional
baseball player and broadcaster

I was trying to wash my face after dinner, but there was no hot water. No big deal. The kids probably used it all up. I'd been in enough hot water for one lifetime to worry about it for an evening.

So I cleared most of the Kabuki Theater sunscreen off with some cold rags, snuck off to the "think tank" I had built off a roof deck, and pulled a few choice literary morsels for the night: Schopenhauer, Updike, a little Rumi for dessert.

"S. T.!" I heard the shriek from the bathroom shower. "There's no hot water." Now with my wife involved in the problem, I was drafted. A trip down to the garage revealed three inches of nice hot water, perfect for a day's-end shower, covering the cement floor. Shit. So much for a nice relaxing evening.

It was a Saturday night and my first thought was to call my good buddy Ray Odell. Ray is a plumber, an electrician, a real-world MacGyver who can fix any broken object that has been given a name.

But I couldn't call Ray, not on a Saturday night. Not even on Sunday. The man had bailed me out of more domestic debacles than I could list on six pages. I'd wait until Monday. We'd be fine without water for a day. At least my son and I would. The girls would take some convincing.

And as I lumbered down to have a look at the hot water heater, I thought of Ray and listened to myself think.

You remember when you first met Ray? When he came to the house and worked on that ridiculous idea you had to build a steam room out of a tiny broom closet?

"Of course. He was...stockier then. Might have smoked too. I don't think he was too athletic. Good plumber though."

No, he wasn't a big jock like your punk ass. But he made some changes, didn't he? You gave him those old shoes because his feet were the same size as yours and you had a damn store-full in your garage didn't you? Remember when he started running? He eventually did a 10K, then a half marathon, and finally that Ironman thing you were so wrapped up in.

"Yeah, Ray went through some heavy life changes—left his job, built up his own business, got divorced, started surfing again, remarried, got fit, fell out of shape, built his own log cabin in the mountains, wrote some songs, got fit again."

The only constant is change, eh?

"Yeah, the world is in motion and even if you try to sit still, something comes along and knocks you off your comfortable center."

You didn't used to talk like that.

"I thought my center was pretty secure."

You have to find your edges to find your center. What about Ray?

"Well, I was just thinking how he never saw a lot of those changes coming, how he must've been like everybody else and figured that all the hard shit would come flying at somebody else."

Like when you were showing off and went flying down that cliff on your mountain bike and broke two vertebrae in your neck?

"Yeah, that was a wake-up call. Had an angel riding shotgun on that trip."

You should be racing wheelchairs with your bud David Bailey.

"I should be dead, considering all the rad stuff I did as a kid."

You should be dead considering all the rad stuff you did as an adult.

"The more things change, the more they stay the same."

So we gonna call Ray to come and fix your hot water heater? Or you gonna try to replace it yourself and mess it up like you did that pool heater? Remember? You were telling your daughter Torrie you could fix anything.

"Yes, I'm gonna call Ray, on Monday. And I can fix most things that are busted, at least the small stuff. Ask Torrie about all the dolls and toys of hers I fixed."

Speaking of change, she's grown up. It's hard to recognize her.

"If you spent more time with her like you did when she was a kid and you and Virginia drug her ass all over the world so you could race…"

She's a teenager. She needs to build her own life, grow up and make it on her own. I don't think she hates me, she just needs the distance right now.

"You love her don't you? Miss doing stuff with her, don't you?"

More than you'll ever know.

"Oh, I know. We're the same aren't we?"

And aren't we talking about loss? The feeling of loss over a daughter growing up, a change in career.

"And losing that hot water heater."

Yeah, but if you called Ray, he wouldn't think twice, he'd be here in thirty minutes, wouldn't he?

"He'd be here in twenty, we'd jury-rig the thing for the night, have a few beers, play a few songs, and my wife would keep me around another week."

So, in everything that you lose, something can be gained.

"One kind of Saturday night for another; one type of relationship with your daughter for another."

…hot water for a friend.

"Good trade."

Reaching

"I can only think of one real reason why I attended my ten-year high school reunion—to rub it in."
—From the author's journal, July 12, 1984

*M*ost really good athletes I know were always good. There are fewer and fewer athletes who make it to the professional level without a past that includes early coaching, parental support, if not pushing, and innate talent. Lots of born-with skills. The level of ability at the top is just too high for a kid to reach unless he has everything going for him. Yeah, Tiger Woods is good because he works hard, but he also had talent, coaching, parental support, proper equipment, and competitive opportunities. Tiger Woods is a golfing example of what it takes to reach the rarified heights of professional sport. It would be unfair, untrue, and cynical to say that all pros succeed because they have been given unusual opportunities to develop their talent. But the fact is, it helps. A lot.

Maybe that's why we love to hear the story of the inner-city kid from the poor family who grew up shooting hundreds of thousands of free throws up at a bent, rusted hoop on an old school yard court with weeds growing up through cracks in the asphalt. You can picture him—a tall, lanky kid in baggy shorts and his older brother's dirty white tank top. He dribbles, shoots, moves, dribbles, shoots, moves, dribbles, shoots, moves. And the light grows dim. He looks around to make sure there are no gangs, no *clicas* gathering on the corner, takes another shot, the sound of sirens wailing in the near distance. Watching the arc of the ball as it leaves his delicate fingertips like a shooting star, he sees it pass cleanly through the rusty orange ring before hearing the metallic swoosh of the metal chain; only because light travels faster than sound. He hears the sound of the crowd as he sees himself in his dreams, making that shot, defying physics.

It's a scene played out in popular films and stories all the time. And we embrace the ideal because it brings our heroes closer to us. It gives them a human past. Most of us know we will never make it to the level where crowds will cheer for our play, but the idea that it is *possible* gives us hope.

I didn't start my career as a poor inner-city youth, but I didn't start it with personal coaching and instructional videos either. In the late '70s, triathlon wasn't a sport, it was an underground cult of multisport enthusiasts—burned-out runners, aging fitness buffs, and skilled lifeguards displaying their many talents. I shared membership in each of those odd athletic categories.

There was no blueprint on how to train. No coaches, camps, clinics, videos, or how-to manuals. It was all trial and error. And a ton of hard work. Most of us were very unsophisticated. But a small group of us knew instinctively that this sport could be something, that its charisma would move out like jungle vines, gathering in first the odd and unkempt, then the risk-takers, and finally the masses. And a few, like myself, held secret hopes that we could ride this wave and retain our squatters' rights on the depth of our willingness to suffer.

The hardest-working athlete in those early years was Scott Molina, a talented kid from the blue-collar town of Pittsburg, California. Scott was one of six kids, the son of a maintenance worker at the Dow Chemical plant and a schoolbus driver. They weren't rich.

The first time I saw Molina was in an outtake from a short documentary on the Ironman being filmed by Rodney Jacobs, a young producer from Aspen, Colorado, a man who has remained a close friend of mine for well over twenty years.

Rodney called me up at our little house in the funky town of Ocean Beach and said he was making a film on the race in Hawaii. It was the first time anybody in the media apart from local reporters had ever contacted me about the sport.

When he and his "crew" (a friend of his who knew how to operate a camera) showed up to interview my brother and me, he told me of this kid up north whom they had just shot and offered to show me a clip. I will never forget what I saw when Rodney plugged the Beta-format videotape into his machine. The soundless footage showed a twenty-two-year-old working as a short-order cook at Kmart during the day and as a stock boy at a liquor store at night and living in a fifteen- by twenty-foot trailer with his young wife and six-month-old baby girl. In between all this, he was training for the Hawaiian Ironman triathlon: swimming before work in the morning, running during his lunch break, and riding his bike in the cold dark after work.

While my schedule wasn't all that different, I did have a good job and a house that I couldn't hook up behind a car and drive away. Something clicked when I witnessed Molina's work ethic; something inside me shifted and bent at an angle where it had previously run straight. There was still no money or professional opportunity in the sport, but there were people who worked harder to win. And at least one who worked harder than I did.

The deeper I looked into my soul, the less I saw of my present self, the grad student, the sailing instructor, and the more I saw of my potential self—the athlete. If I were going to take a shot at this sport, money or not, I would have to fashion and wear my own crown of thorns. And prove to the memory of my dad that I could be a good athlete. Maybe even a great one.

> *"All these prima donnas, who do they think they are, walking around like they are more special than the rest of us. They're being paid millions of bucks and they still want more. Geez, let them come and work a regular job for a while. They might appreciate what they got more."*
>
> —Anonymous fan on the
> state of professional
> athlete salaries

▼ ▼ ▼

Sometimes we fail our heroes because they fail us. They don't fit into the mold we need them to; the relationship isn't there. Or if it is, it is one of mutual disdain.

No one can fault Scott Molina for doing all that he could. He had the same motivation we all did—to better his life. Becoming a hero was the furthest thing from our minds. But a better lifestyle, doing something we loved, something we were compelled to do, something without which our lives would seem impoverished—that was the motivation. As Sly Stallone said in *Rocky III*, "Men like us don't have a choice."

Molina and I became close friends over the years, and every time I visit Jacobs in his studio I ask him to find that old footage of a twenty-two-year-old Molina making hamburgers in a grease-stained cook's outfit, glancing at the clock, wondering what kind of running workout he'd get in on his break.

"I had a feeling," Molina remembers, "that triathlon might take off, might get noticed by the public, the media, and some money would be offered in prizes and sponsorship. If that happened, I was going to be ready."

When the 1982 Ironman came around in a few months, he wasn't there and he wasn't ready, the victim of a bike accident. Molina was riding home from Dave's Liquor late at night and decided to take a detour, you know, add a few extra miles before arriving at his metal box lined up with dozens of other trailers in the RV park. A car drifted to the shoulder and edged Scott off into the ditch.

He would be okay, but he missed the biggest race in the sport, an event that drew just over three hundred athletes, huge by triathlon standards. And all that film of him flipping meat patties for the customers while they went off in search of twenty-four-ounce jars of peanut butter and twelve-packs of Coke would be wasted. But he would heal and train harder, maybe add an extra light to the back of his bike.

When athletes from humble beginnings make it to the pros, two things can happen. They may remember their roots, keep their egos in check, and buy their mamma a house in a new suburb. Or they may forget all that and revel in their newfound success, accept the adulation and internalize it, make it part of the *new them*, the pro athlete.

Few are the anecdotes of men and women who fell in between, who appreciated what they had achieved, who tasted a bite or two of the forbidden fruit, but who never really believed the idolizing sound bytes on the news.

After I won the Ironman in February 1982 and returned home to my job, everything seemed anticlimactic. In the days and weeks after the event, what I had accomplished just wouldn't set in. I got stuck between worlds: I was a surf-bum sailing instructor taking a few classes, feeling society's pressure to grow up, go corporate, cut my hair, or at least buy a pair of long pants, and at the same time I felt a powerful draw toward the ethereal realm of world-class sport. I was terribly conflicted and, in true Tinley fashion, I tried to do it all. I did my job on Mission Bay in San Diego and went out drinking a few nights a week after work with the mostly young and single instructors who worked under me; then I raced home and ran for an hour, half the time with a good buzz; then I drove out to school for a night class, getting home at 11 P.M.; and then I got up early to sneak in a swim before starting work again. As you can imagine, my new wife wasn't thrilled with this pattern of behavior, and to this day I think she still remembers that crazy-ass first year of our marriage as a dark time, which the years since have not washed clean.

As for the rest of the sporting world, winning the Ironman in 1982 was simply no big deal. Ironically, that was my good fortune. Soon enough they would know of this sport, and people would come calling. And I would have to make harder choices, both in who I was and where I was going.

The Lure of the Gold

"My dad was my biggest hero, but they haven't made a poster of him yet."
— Derek Jeter, professional baseball player

B ehind every great athlete is a drive to succeed—a drive empowered by a goal, pushed by a dream, embedded in a quest. The choices these men and women make along the way reflect their dreams and their quests. But underneath it all, most athletes love the game. Almost all athletes who reach top levels experience enormous pleasure in simply doing the activity itself, regardless of other motivations and benefits. You have to love what you're doing.

There are great benefits to hitting the "bigs," to making the "show." Everybody knows what they are, everybody wants them. There is gold in them thar hills. All you have to do is become one of the best athletes in the world at any given sport, seize the opportunity to prove it when it counts the most—when everybody is watching, when everybody needs somebody like you—and then hang on for the ride. That's all. And it all starts when you're a kid, when you do it for fun.

"Every day when I drive home," says Antawn Jamison, forward for the Golden State Warriors, "there is a basketball court there, and sometimes I'll just pull over and see how the kids are playing the game. It brings back memories of me out there."

The dream almost always begins here, when the developing child's identity melds into the athlete's identity. Very few athletes decide in their mid or late twenties to shoot for the top. The levels of competition are just too high. The mindset of the athlete emerges in youth, when the metal is hot, when critical choices are made, when the framework for one's life is built.

Tim Flannery, former utility player and third base coach for the San Diego Padres, grew up in Orange County, California, right down the street from Anaheim Stadium, home of the Anaheim Angels and the Big A, a five-story neon sign, one of the first giant totems used by pro teams to create identity with the fans. Tim recalls those days playing Little League baseball, then seniors, and then the Babe Ruth League: "Every day I would drive by that big A out in front of the stadium, and if the team won I'd see all the neon lights flashing like some great City of Oz. I was drawn to it like a giant magnet and all that it stood for."

When Flannery made the Show, he became a symbol for all that it takes: He was the lion receiving courage from the wizard, and a real-world testimony to the dream at work. Whenever I took my son and his buddies to a Padres game, we would sneak down from the nosebleed seats to the third base line between innings and try to get Flannery's attention.

"Hey what's up Tinley?" he'd call out. "You ride your bike up to Los Angeles and back today?" And my kid and his buddies and the people sitting in the expensive seats would think more highly of me because I happened to know a third base coach and he'd joked with me. These little things make you a little part of the dream.

Many of these dreams originate in myths or legends that pass from parent to child through stories, folklore, literature, or pure symbols, like a giant neon A. And they contain elements of desire; they are unpredictable and are developed from realizations that they have messages in a symbolic form. We may not know it at the time but the stories develop or awaken a sleeping need to excel, to do something of significance with our lives. The hidden symbols can be in our memories of the way our parents showed us love and care in their storytelling or something more obtuse, and distant, like a particular place or character that resonates powerfully within our psyche; we rarely know why, but we don't forget either.

▼ ▼ ▼

After my career began to take off in 1983, a friend approached me about teaming up with him and a few other businessmen to start a performance clothing line. Sure, I told him, I'd be happy to wear the product, test it out, provide some feedback. Heck, he was even going to pay me for it.

Within eighteen months the company had my name on it and I was an equity shareholder. My partners and the growing cadre of employees covered the day-to-day duties; all I had to do was keep training my ass off to remain near the top of the sport. On a good week, I'd even fulfill my marketing and promotion duties. But they weren't that taxing and, hell, I was going to be the best athlete I could be anyway.

The product was a hit and now the Tinley logo would be emblazoned across the chests and backs of runners and triathletes everywhere. Suddenly I appeared to be a more talented athlete because I had a clothing line with my name on it. I never would have predicted it. The decision was a business move—buyers would imagine my wife sewing little running shorts while I packed them in cardboard boxes and shipped them off between workouts. Everybody loves a mom-and-pop success story.

Actually I was embarrassed by it all and the fame it brought me. The consumer took part in the myth by wearing a bathing suit with a symbol, the athlete's name, printed down the side. And that name was mine. One of the first times I saw another athlete wearing a pair of Tinley bike shorts with the family name screened down the left leg, I was with my friend and training partner Vic Rosenthal.

"Did you see that?" he screamed. "Did you? I can't fucking believe it. You're a superstar, you asshole, a bona fide icon. Geez, now I've seen everything—an average-skilled-jock-surf bum with his name on someone else's ass."

It was uncomfortable to see my name on the side of a building, and a balloon in my caricatured likeness that could have been entered in the Macy's Thanksgiving Day Parade. I went from being one of the guys trying to make it to an image, a marketing vehicle, and at times a target. Suddenly I was reading about myself in the papers and I was "recognizable" within the small circles of multisport competition. It was...weird. But the money was nice. We went from "getting by" to being able to pick up the tab for a group dinner without thinking about which event I'd have to win to pay for it. My wife now worked for the company and we could afford a child and a new house. At twenty-six I bought my first new car, a base model Saab 900 that had bicycle chain grease on the suede seats within two days. It was way too yuppie for me, and I sold it after six months and bought my wife an SUV and myself an older pickup truck. But now I could afford one with four-wheel drive. As far as I was concerned, it couldn't get any better.

By becoming a top athlete you also become a symbol of many things, both good and evil, that we all desire: strength, power, grace, control, acclaim, money, fame, opportunity, respect, self-esteem, and immortality. And in some respects, whether real or perceived, you represent a *higher* form of living. Being a partner in a company that made running shorts in a flowery print only elevated my *sense* of living. But for me to justify the commodification of my success, I had to work out even harder, and win even more. If I didn't do well, I'd feel even more guilt about all my partners and the employees having to work long days while I rode my bike out in the sun. Back then, this sense of higher living had to be grounded in the reality of race victories.

I ran into an old friend and coach named Steve Estes one day. Steve is a former national rowing team member and currently a professor of physical education at East Carolina University. He has followed a path I aspire to at times—from the ultimate physical challenge of elite sports to the ultimate cerebral quest of an intellectual life. Not many achieve it. He knew very well what I had experienced and I latched onto him, sending him drafts of papers I would write on various studies within the sociology and psychology of sport.

"There is a critical point to your study of athletes," he mused over a couple of beers one night. "You people, the athletes yourselves, *live* in the most profound way that the word can be used. It is the *life* of the athlete that is critical. The 'professional' moniker is just the explicit, observable trappings of a way of living."

Ultimately, I knew he was right. Maybe that sense of heightened existence overshadows all the other perks that we assume will come with a successful sporting life—the thought that all you have to do is win one major title, one championship, and everything in your life after that will be an easy ride. It's become cliché, but I've found it to be one of the great truisms in my life: The rewards come during the journey, when you do everything you can to feel and embrace life, even the pain and suffering. Athletes who are naturally concerned with the next game, the next workout, or the next season lose the ability to feel alive in the moment of competition—when their bodies are young and limber, when the afternoon sky is filled with the sound of the fans and the smell of fresh-cut grass, when they're just anxious enough to be ready for the next race or inning or quarter. That's when it doesn't get any better. That's when you get paid for all your hard work. The reward comes in the form of indelible memories, which no one can ever take away from you. That's why you're an athlete.

There are any number of psychologists who will tell you that sport is a substitute for war, that it enables the athlete, especially the male athlete, to discharge aggression and a corresponding machismo, all innocuously under the guise of competition. And just like war movies, competition sells.

After I won that first Ironman in 1982, I had barely made it back to the hotel after the race when some guy from Los Angeles called to invite me to be a participant in a made-for-TV outdoor-oriented event called Survival of the Fittest. Not being a real sports fan or a TV watcher, I wasn't sure what it was. But the offer included an all-expense-paid trip to New Zealand and a chance to compete in a unique series of events that ranged from whitewater kayaking, to climbing and rappelling, to jousting on a narrow bridge thirty feet over a crystal-clear river. I would have had to save up for five years to take a trip like that, and here was some voice trying to convince me I should go because it would be on national television. I didn't give a shit about the TV. I just couldn't get over the idea that they wanted me to be a contestant. All I had done was finish first in a swim-bike-run race with five hundred people in it. The prize I won was an eighteen-inch koa wood trophy, a cool-looking piece of wood and one of the only trophies I still own.

Sign me up dude. When do we leave? I was ready to be challenged, to see if I could "survive." But mostly I was thinking about seeing the world on someone else's meal ticket.

A month later I was in a little town on the South Island of New Zealand with a collection of mountain goat freaks who could do pull-ups with one finger at a time and scale any sheer wall we passed by. They were serious about this stuff. For them, it was a coveted title, a bragging-rights kind of thing. I was at a vacation race; they were at war.

No one can say if making war is an innate trait in the human species. And maybe sport's greatest gift to the world is the substitute of defeat for death. And that's a good thing. Because in Survival of the Fittest, I was getting *killed* in every event. One day they flew us to the top of a steep, rocky mountain, lined us up shoulder to shoulder, turned the cameras on, and told us to race to the bottom. Most of the guys were clad in warrior garb—helmets, pads, gloves, and testosterone. All I wanted to do was get down the mountain without breaking anything and keep all my blood inside my body where it belonged. I had won the Ironman; I had finally convinced myself that I didn't have anything to prove. Still, when the gun was fired, I forgot all that.

Mankind is drawn to the great physical challenge of domination. Not too many generations ago, some of this desire was channeled into the basic challenge of surviving, of providing food and shelter for oneself and one's family. But even if you worked fourteen hours out in the field, you could still find the energy to go running around with knives and guns and arrows, looking to claim what is yours, or to keep out those who say it's theirs. Maybe it was food, maybe it was land. In the world of sport, it's a trophy and a paycheck.

Some sublimate this drive into business ventures, hoping that the world of commerce will provide a playing field on which they can succeed. Others turn to breaking the law, or anti-social rebelliousness. But sports, ah sports, offers acceptable forms of battle and domination. If there isn't a "battle" to be fought in your life, no matter—the local sport magazines are filled with race applications.

When I got to the bottom of the hill, I was cut, scraped, and bruised, but nothing was broken. Two of the competitors who finished in front of me had managed to crack something. Tough luck, I thought. It's going to be hard for them to manage the upcoming obstacle course in casts.

Around this time I was noticing a change in myself that was not entirely positive. I felt very proud of my accomplishments but I was slowly getting sucked into that thick fog of high-level sport, where stale sweat mixes with sweet perfume. I had been given one more taste of the bennies of success. I had never considered myself a fighter, but it sure felt good to win battles. My world seemed dreamlike, a Valhalla. And the dream pried my body out of bed at 5:30 in the morning to run twelve miles when my blood alcohol was still .10, or I had been up working on a paper until 3 A.M.

I was no hero because everybody around me knew me for what I was: a young man trying to find my way in life, switching jobs, desperately trying to avoid one that would put my sandy feet under a desk.

But now I knew the taste of the hero's life. And in the ordinary hours it too pulled me like the earth's gravity.

It's hard to know when you should give sport your all, when you should make it your companion, your lover, and your life. The lure of fame gets in the way; your heart gets in the way. Objectivity be damned. It's hard to be really honest with yourself when you're trying so hard to let the truth in. Or maybe if you can be objective in hindsight, like John McEnroe, you will someday realize that you weren't really sure.

"Sometimes, when I look back, I don't know how any of this ever happened to me," he remembers. "The truth is, I didn't really want to pursue tennis, until it just pursued me."

Behind that pursuit is often a prodding, pushing parent, not always looking out for the child's best interest. When you listen to top athletes talk about their childhoods, you often hear a distaste for the pressure and meddling they experienced growing up, regardless of the advantages they have gained from sport. Common remarks:

"I hated swimming for years."

"I wanted to quit gymnastics so bad. They starved me for six years!"

"I only played because my parents wanted that scholarship for me so bad. I would have quit football after high school."

It is hard to imagine a more grotesque story of parental involvement in sports than the recent case in which an enraged father beat to death the coach of his child's hockey team.

Nonetheless, when the scholarships, Olympic medals, and pro contracts are handed out, who do the players thank first? Their parents. And when you see that you have a chance at the big time? You take it. Tomorrow can be dealt with tomorrow.

This is one of the unique paradoxes of athletic greatness. To reach your potential in most sports, you must defer the typical maturation process and focus solely on developing as an athlete. You know that you only get one shot. You have to take it.

Years later, if you're lucky, it will all come into perspective. But you don't get to pick the time. And the fall off the back can be harder than the climb to the top.

After the last event in the Survival of the Fittest contest was run and the scores were tallied, I hadn't finished last but I was damn close. The only other triathlete in the competition was a woman named Julie Moss, a perky young redhead who had crawled across the finish line and into the annals of sporting history with her dramatic second-place finish in the 1982 Ironman. It was the same event which I had just won a few months before and her showing had also earned her a trip to the Survival event in New Zealand, where she finished last. We triathletes had made a strong statement about our fledgling sport. We were pretty good—at going in a straight line with no geographical obstacles.

▼ ▼ ▼

As I sat at the only bar in the tiny town of Wanaka, New Zealand, that night, a bit embarrassed by my performance, I was approached by an older man smoking a huge cigar and wearing an even bigger New York-style smile.

"Hi Scott," he said over the raucous background. "Did you enjoy yourself? Pretty wild event we got here, isn't it? Name's Barry Frank. I sort of put this whole thing together. Hey, let me get you another beer."

"Well, yes Barry, it's quite different than triathlons."

"Listen Scott," he glanced around the room as if seeking spying ears. "I think you guys have something with this new sport of yours. I want to hire you to help me put on the biggest and best triathlon in the world. I'm thinking Europe, maybe Monaco. We have an office over there and good connections with the locals. Can you fly over there in a few weeks and set up a course?"

I'd never even been to Europe, and in a singular moment I had been approached by one of the most powerful men in sports entertainment about flying first-class to Monte Carlo to consult on the development of what would become one of the most prestigious triathlons in the world.

I accepted the fresh beer, told him I was all ears, and began formulating excuses in my mind to scam yet another week off of work.

How Hard, How Bad?
Costs, Rewards,
and Questions

*W*hen I'm asked about my career in sport, these are the things that come into my mind first:

1. Good friends
2. Seeing the world
3. Having the chance to be "different"
4. Meeting interesting people
5. Hard work
6. My kids bragging about me
7. The rest of my friends

These are the things I don't think about:

1. Winning races
2. How good I was
3. Having been a pioneer in a new sport
4. Wishing I could do it again
5. Wondering if I could have trained smarter
6. What did I learn?

These are the things I should think more about:

1. How lucky I was
2. Was I self-centered and narcissistic?
3. How did my career affect my family?
4. How much fun I had with my friends
5. What did I learn?

A few people are born to excel in ways large and small that most never experience. Most never feel the false warmth and the abrasive glare of the media lights. For those who desire to excel at sport, to develop their typically inborn physical gifts into a skill that sets them in a class with a few hundred others in the world, hard work is the key.

Their dues are paid in a literal sweat equity that opens the first of so many doors one must get through to get *there*. At this level, the workload is almost surreal. I have seen many professional and Olympic athletes cry in pain at some point. To train at the world-class level is more than a verb. It is a quest toward the possibilities, the substance behind the battle to excel.

To get paid to race in a sport that I had previously paid to compete in, well, that was the ultimate carrot dangling in my unsure future. It wasn't as if the money was huge. And I had been raised knowing that money did not buy happiness, especially since we didn't have much—money, that is. I knew this, though, after getting a job boxing groceries at age fifteen: A few bucks sure could blunt some of life's sharper edges.

With the advent of a few prize money races in the summer of 1982, my outlook began to change. The first race with prize money I entered paid $500 for first place, $300 for second, and $200 for the third-place finish I took back to my job at the Mission Bay Aquatic Center. The triathlon lasted just under three hours; my job paid about $250 per week for close to fifty hours of what could loosely be called "work." It was a Disneyland of sailing, surfing, waterskiing, and paddling, with all the trappings of teaching college kids these aquatic pleasures. I considered it one of the best jobs on the planet, even though my recent marriage was tested by the Center's wonderful atmosphere of debauchery.

But I had never forgotten what it felt like to *matter*. The money was a nice carrot. But I had won the biggest race in the sport back in February and hadn't made a dime from it. No, I take that back. I was receiving up to three pairs of free shoes per year and a few warm-up suits in return for wearing a rather large logo on the chest of my racing uniform. There was something else drawing this moth to the flame. Some lure.

But this call I heard was still vague, a strange combination of desire, need, and fulfillment. My friends and coworkers didn't understand my increasing exercise load. Someone else's life is almost always a mystery, just as it can be to that individual himself. At twenty-six years old, who the hell knows what he or she is all about? But I knew there were *opportunities*. I decided that if I was going to have a go at this new sport, I would have to work harder, train longer, with more intensity, and more ambition, blind though it may have been. On my longer runs of twenty or twenty-five miles, I would debate my plans with myself.

So, you want to be a superstar, eh hotshot?

"No, I just want a shot. I want to see what I can do."

Well what's so bad about getting a regular job, raising a few regular kids, waxing the Volvo on Saturday, and watching the game on Sunday?

"Nothing. It's just that I feel like I've been called to take this shot, to sacrifice the leather interior and the big screen to see if I can make it in the Game."

Well, I suppose that sometimes in life a part of that life chooses us, not the other way around. But remember, if you make it in the Game, in the end you may only have the Game.

Once young athletes smell success in sport, once they get a taste of high-level achievement—when they can look in the mirror and know without saying it that they are good, very very good—the sport becomes their rock. It is the foundation on which all elements of their

lives are built, the planet around which other duties and responsibilities revolve. And they will break themselves against that rock to
make it to the top of the pile.

Former NFL player Jessie Tuggle once said about his relationship
to the game, "Throughout my whole career, I've worked as hard as I
can to be the best I can be. It's sort of funny, from the outside looking
in, the average fan would think it's the money that motivates me. It's
not. On Sundays, you don't think about that...It's a privilege to play
in this league."

I wanted that "privilege" and I knew it was rooted in work, in
training harder than you ever thought possible. The suffering was hell
at times but from the little success that I had experienced, the privilege felt like grace.

I was entering that place in an athlete's life where the only certainty is overwhelming ambiguity. You might think that "turning pro"
would simplify your life—that there would be fewer distractions,
fewer gray areas, and the clear goal of doing all that is physically and
mentally possible to reach the top of the pile. In truth it does not. You
still live in a fog of subjectivity that blurs the lines of reality and
clouds your judgment. The only thing that counts is your training and
competing. Nothing else fits. And you become that which you think
about: an athlete.

When I first had the notion that triathlon could, at some point in
the near future, provide a degree of financial opportunity, something
inside me clicked. I was like every young boy who dreams of being a
pro athlete, only now, in the summer of 1982, there were a few signs
that this might actually be a possibility. I started doing the math. How
many wins? How much prize money? What about travel costs, house
payments, food, car expenses, my wife's job?

Those were only numbers, though. The reality of a regular life
might be lost in the rising vapor of illusion and the clarity of my future direction losing its way in the Dream but I had a shot at being a
pro athlete, of getting paid to play, of being my own boss, of walking
away from all the old rules.

You don't walk away from that.

The rebel heart inside me beat louder to the Dream, the Dream of telling the world that I would live on my own terms, of making a difference. Of course, this idealistic combination of Henry David Thoreau and James Dean was entirely impractical—which made it only more attractive. If I were a hero, living a life of significance again, the hidden challenges of my past would get absorbed in the miles and the travel and the victory celebrations. Who can ever compare their childhood experiences against the yardstick of adult success without second guessing the past and risking the present? I was lucky to grow up in a big family with great parents, grandparents, aunts and uncles, and friends. We didn't go hungry; we got two new pairs of shoes every year. But something must have affected me significantly; something profound and unnamed must have crawled under my thin ten-year-old skin and lay dormant, waiting for a chance to break up and shout, "Look at me! I can climb that tree. I can build that fort. I can do it. And everybody who needs a home can come and hang out. Just you watch. My fort will be higher and different than any fort you've ever seen." If I were a professional athlete, my life would *matter* again. I could make a difference, if only in my own mind. All it would take would be work. And triathlon was a perfect tree. So I put my head down and went to work. For twenty years.

Viktor Frankl wrote in *Man's Search for Meaning* that "suffering ceases to be suffering at the moment it finds meaning." My training felt like suffering many times. I had no compass to follow, no map or training program or coach or guidelines. In the early days of triathlon we were all lab rats in search of the perfect training program. If two hundred miles per week was good, then three hundred was better, and four hundred better yet.

I'd get up in the morning and roll down the driveway on my bike, waving at my neighbors who were headed off to work at the office. On the really long days, I'd come peddling back up the driveway at about the same time they were returning from their jobs, each of us having put in a full day. It was work, I told myself, plain, simple, and hard. Miles in the bank, to be withdrawn on race day. In that sense, eight hours of sitting on a three-inch wide bike seat pushing those damn pedals took on meaning. My suffering had a purpose behind it. But it still felt like suffering.

There were days when I knew I would be better off taking it easy or resting altogether. A little moderation would have given my body the rest it was craving and would have made me a better athlete over-all. In my mind I knew this. Still, I couldn't help myself: I was ad-dicted to the feeling that the training gave me, the sense of freedom, of self-reliance, the constant reinforcement of my faith that I could tell the corporate world it wouldn't put leather shoes on my feet and screw me to a desk—I was a pro athlete, a rebel who needed no cause. I raced for myself and a few loyal sponsors. Because I could.

In races when the going was particularly hard, I pondered where this ability to suffer came from. I certainly didn't enjoy it. I was inter-ested in the benefits—the outward ones like money, the inward ones like self-knowledge. What was driving me anyway? I wanted to know so I could nurture it, keep it going as long as I could. I have never an-swered that question. I suspect it had its root in guilt, maybe over my father's early death, or some inherent need to be the best at a game of my own choosing. Maybe I just craved the attention and disguised myself as an iconoclastic loner. I may never know.

Looking back into that rearview mirror, that reflective piece of my life that lay exposed, a physical Babylon begging to be found and fondled, I think often of the work. In fact, few things enter my conscience before the long, sometimes lonely miles do. Not the money, the perks, the applause, none of the inconsequential results that seem shallow and materialistic in hindsight. I remember them; can't deny the tangible benefits of a successful career, but what I like to recall are stories like this; tales that illustrate what did matter in the end.

I once interviewed the ageless fitness guru Jack LaLanne. Having always admired his work ethic, and wanting to speak to him, I spent months wending through his protective wall of PR people. In the end it was a quote of his own from an old *Outside Magazine* article that got me an audience with a man closing in on eighty years old at the time: "Ask the guys who are doing serious triathlons if there are limits to what can be done," he had said. And then, pointing to his own head hiding beneath red curly hair, "The limit is right here."

When I finally met the man who had been a fitness fixture on American television for almost forty years, he was asleep, just lying there on a big cushy chair with his feet propped up on the footrest and the TV blaring a sports show in the background. On the phone his wife had told me to "let myself in" if Jack didn't get to the door right away. I knocked and pounded and rang and called out for almost twenty minutes before cracking the door and calling out softly, "Oh Mr. LaLanne?" Hearing the TV I crept upstairs, terrified that he was going to think I was an intruder and put a round from a rusty thirty-aught-six right through my leg.

Here was one of the greatest fitness specimens to grace the human race, lying down. And for just the slightest of moments, when I saw him swallowed up in the old lounge chair, mouth slightly ajar, I thought he was dead. Irony raced from synapse to synapse. Nothing could kill this man. He was destined to live forever. As he has said on many occasions, "I can't die. It would ruin my image." What if I frightened him into a heart attack? I might as well go look for that gun and end my own life.

Then Jack bolted up like a spring-loaded jackknife.

"Where you been hotshot? You were supposed to be here an hour ago. We have work to do."

"Work?" I asked. "Don't you need to warm up? We can talk a bit."

"Ever see a lion warm up before he goes for an antelope? Let me show you the gym, my temple. We'll see how fit you are."

And that's how it went, two old dogs, one twice the age of the other, not so much comparing notes as sharing what they knew and what they had done by working out together.

I wanted to ask Jack about pain tolerance in athletes and about a study I had read comparing groups of athletes and non-athletes. The study showed that athletes who participated in a contact sport had, on average, a pain tolerance 40% higher than non-athletes; athletes in non-contact sports had a pain tolerance 20% higher. But I knew the question would not interest a man like LaLanne.

At one point, after Jack had warmed to me a bit, and introduced me to his wife and dog, he put me in his pool and showed me his secret butterfly stroke.

"This is how I pulled seventy-six people in thirteen rowboats on the country's bicentennial. Did it handcuffed too. Try that hotshot. Makes the Ironman look like a 5K."

I did, and he was right. But what I walked away with at the end of the day, besides absolute admiration for this sage and new friend, was a new appreciation of the fact that if you want to be the best you can be, and you want to maintain or improve that level of fitness, you work very, very hard, rest on a comfortable chair for awhile, and then work some more.

How much is enough? You know it's something special to make it all the way to the top. Hell, if every kid could play in the pros, it wouldn't mean that much, would it? And most of us have been socialized believing, *knowing* that all heroes work hard.

Robin Hood would shoot hundreds of arrows a day in practice, Luke Skywalker worked his light saber, Ulysses wrestled, Rocky jogged through a pre-dawn Philadelphia ghetto. And if all things come together, and we make the Big Leagues, the hard work pays off. Our suffering really did have meaning. And in hindsight, it doesn't seem so bad.

I remember one spring day at the peak of my career when I was training so hard that I was constantly dead tired. My muscles were sore to the touch. We were doing a long swim set, something like six repeats of five hundred yards, and somewhere near the middle of the fifth one I fell asleep while swimming. I swear it's true. I went ten or fifteen yards, hit the wall with my hand, and woke up scared. In my heart of hearts, I knew I was close to the edge of something other than the pool. But the adrenaline of the experience pushed me through the last five hundred yards, and I just kept hammering away at my body, like a man digging his own grave, like a bat hanging upside down in the daylight, not because I had a death wish but because the draw of success was so powerful, because my buddies were right there next to me, because I was doing what I thought I was born to do.

The cold, hard fact is that no matter how hard they work, professional athletes actually play professional sports for somewhere between six and seven years, on average, and much less than that in certain sports like pro football. One must wonder if all that work is worth it. Rare is the athlete who does.

Even if we know that our lives after sports won't have the same meaning, still we push on, figuring out how we can improve, how we can win next week, or next year, never considering that it might end soon—because how could it? I just worked my ass off for ten years to get here!

John Ed Bradley, a former offensive lineman for LSU and now a successful writer, once said in an article for *Sports Illustrated*: "I was only twenty-one years old, yet I believed that nothing I did for the rest of my life would rise up to those days when I wore the Purple and Gold. I might go on to make a lot of money, I might marry a beautiful woman and fill a house with perfect kids. I might make a mark that would be significant in other people's eyes. But I would never have it better than when I played football for LSU."

He claims, and I believe him, that there was a time when he considered drafting a stipulation that he be buried in an old rotting T-shirt declaring in black letters: "Nobody Works Harder Than the Offensive Line."

Making the Show

"Sometimes you go to funerals and sometimes you go to weddings. And to me this is a party."
—Wayne Gretzky, at Madison Square Garden
announcing his retirement

*I*n sports, where everything, including the player, is in a state of flux, you get the feeling that if something doesn't happen, trouble sets in. So it is for the athlete, who must continually work at his craft until he can improve no more. And then he must fight to retain what age and injury and all the vicissitudes of time's march conspire to take from him.

But there are landmarks along the way, jumping-off places of such significance that they live in an athlete's memory like a testimony to his or her very being. A lifelong player will remember that first touchdown he scored as a high school senior, or the first college tennis match she won, when her parents were there and the coach was smiling. Some carry these images around in their heads alongside their memories of weddings, births, and funerals.

Making the Show, finally getting picked up by a team, or landing a name sponsor is a big thing for an athlete. How he deals with such a life-altering event is an indication of how he'll make the transition back to everyday life, cutting the lawn on Sunday instead of playing on one manicured by professional groundskeepers.

Rare are the humble athletes who don't allow the adulation and ego-boosting to affect their true selves. Self-centered athletes live out their careers in a trite, self-fulfilling prophecy. They think they deserve what they get. And that is true. They deserve all of what they get, long after they are getting nothing. When the good ones make it all the way to the top, it can be the beginning of a morality battle royale. There are so many temptations—not all of them bad—and choices have to be made. But first you have to make it.

Stanford basketball player Casey Jacobsen once said, "When little boys and girls ask me for an autograph...I remember when I was young, how cool the college players were. I wanted to be like them and play like them. Now that I am one, I don't want to forget what it is like to be a child with dreams."

A mature attitude like Jacobsen's appears to stem from how the athlete perceives himself. Athletes are not gods; they are not infallible, seventy home runs in a season or not. They make the same mistakes as everyone else, maybe more. But if an athlete is playing well and the sportswriters can't say enough nice things, it's easy to start believing them.

In the summer of 1984 I went to my ten-year high school reunion. My first year as a competing pro had been as exciting as Mr. Toad's Wild Ride, and the reunion was appropriately held at the Disneyland Hotel in Anaheim, California, right down the street from the Big A. I had debated whether or not to go, mostly because I had only kept in touch with one friend from high school, an old surf buddy named Don Foss who I'd call once or twice a year. My high school years had been swallowed by the mediocrity in which I had passed through them. I had been a mediocre student, a mediocre athlete, and worst of all a mediocre friend. It seemed to me that I had tried to rise above the average, but every time I did I got shot down. I found a subject I really liked—writing—but my English class only spent two weeks on it before moving on to grammar and punctuation. As a junior I was one of the best runners on the cross-country team. Just before my senior season I suffered a stress fracture that kept me out of the lineup; it was two years before I ran well again. I had a crush on a cute little blonde but she had no interest in me; my face broke out in pimples; I had braces put on my crooked teeth. I was a little skinny guy going to a parochial school that was enamored with, funded by, and totally ensconced in its football program. Most of my buddies were on the football team, and they were good guys, but as a non-football player I could never make it into the inner circle.

Midway through my senior year, I said "Fuck this." I wasn't getting an education, I wasn't dating anyone, I wasn't on a team or in a club, my grades weren't good enough to get me into a four-year college, and my shrinking circle of friends was succeeding at all of the above. And my dad was dead.

What I had, though, was a job as a box boy at a supermarket, a beat-up 1967 VW Bug, and resolve. One Sunday I went to church with my mom, something that I had more or less given up on, and threw up a desperation prayer: What the hell I should do? Because I was miserable.

As we walked out of church my mother turned to me and said, "It's a shame that you didn't get to surf more with your dad when he was alive."

My dad had just solved my problem. He told me to go surfing.

After that Sunday, I was no longer a shitty student, an injured runner, or a lost fatherless teenager—I was a surfer. I began cutting school in the mornings, reaping the early glass, and showing up late two or three mornings a week with a forged note from my mom. The school was lenient because they knew of my dad's passing and, if I didn't screw up too bad, I too would pass all my classes and graduate within a few months.

But somebody ratted on me, a big football player I cynically imagined, and the Dean of Boys called me into his office.

"Take off your shoes young man."

"Excuse me, sir?"

"Take off your shoes and spread your toes."

Thinking this was some weird health test, I peeled down my sockless Chuck Taylors to reveal three or four teaspoons of beach sand.

"How does one have sandy feet at ten in the morning, Mr. Tinley?"

"Uh, left over from the weekend sir?"

"It's Thursday son. I'm calling your mother."

And that was it. From then on, I was relegated to after-school wind chop and weekends.

But surfing gave me an identity, a direction, and a vehicle to exercise an independent, searching soul. I was a sixth-generation Californian and surfing was a bridge to my past, a connection to my dad. Floating alone on the cold, uncrowded waves of the early '70s, I felt something profound and essential, a piece of a world I could not label.

Along with two sixteen-ounce Budweisers, my ability to be alone and happy on the ocean gave me the confidence to ask out a girl I had known and admired since fourth grade. Lisa Hecker became my first true girlfriend and, besides my wife, the only woman I'd been completely and totally in love with. She was everything that I wasn't: patient, caring, quiet, smart, and happy in her own skin. It lasted three years; in the end I broke it off and went away to college. One of the things I remember telling her as she cried was that she wasn't athletic enough for me. She looked at me queerly as if to say, what the hell does *that* mean? For it meant nothing to her. How could it? In a scene where there was hardly a right thing to say, I had unknowingly attacked her because she wasn't something that I aspired to be.

From time to time I wondered what happened to Lisa Hecker, and maybe that's what drove me to the reunion, not because I wanted to rekindle any flame (we were both married then) but because I wanted to see how she, and every high school football star, would react to what we all had become. And with any luck, each of us growing into what we were supposed to be.

Of course, I arrived late and then sat in the lobby bar drinking soda waters until I knew everybody else would be drunk enough to tell me the truth, and I would be ready to respond in kind. Walking into the room, I thought I had gotten lost and stumbled into a regional Moose Lodge convention. A quick recon told me what I had suspected: Many of the people I knew had hit their peak early; only a few were aging well. I looked into the eyes of the former cheerleaders and prom queens and heard the words of the Janis Ian song, "At Seventeen": They had "married young and then retired."

It was a strange moment. I had lost my sense of past realities long ago, buried that mediocrity under the ground that I pounded in training, day after day. People whose names I couldn't remember kept coming up to me and relating the most bizarre stories about their "discovery" that I was now a successful professional athlete. I was in a fog of ambivalence when the star fullback or halfback or something-back pulled me aside and said he *had* to buy me a drink.

"Dammit Tinley," he slurred, "there I was sitting on the john taking a dump one Sunday afternoon and in the background I heard your name on the TV and told myself 'I know that skinny punk.' So I did a speed-wipe and watched that whole Ironman Triathlon show from start to finish. Missed the Rams game altogether. Couldn't fucking believe it, kid like you on the tube."

I had lost all sense of objectivity. I needed to leave, but they were giving out awards and I heard my name through the haze: Most Something-or-other. It didn't matter. It was a nice gesture and I appreciated it. I think.

On the way out, somebody tried to sell me life insurance, somebody said I had gotten lucky, and somebody asked me if I wanted to race around the hotel for $50. Then a girl I had dated only once gave me her phone number on a little piece of paper. I stopped and looked at her longer and deeper than I should have, trying to meld the past with the present, chaos with beauty, innocence with responsibility.

"We live just up the coast a bit. My husband would love to meet you. He's a great golfer, you know."

Just before the exit I ran into Lisa Hecker. The long brown hair and engaging brown eyes were still there, buried beneath the thirty-odd pounds she'd added. Her father had died recently and I'd missed the funeral while racing in Japan or Brazil or France. It didn't matter—I wasn't there.

"How's your mother?" I asked.

"You never liked my parents."

"Sure I did. I just didn't know how to show people that I did."

Nothing I could do or say would make a difference to the past or the present. And only the truth would help the future. But at that moment, along with everything else, I couldn't find it.

"I'll see you in ten years at the twentieth reunion, huh?"

Lisa Hecker wasn't at our twentieth reunion in 1994. Nobody tried to sell me anything, nobody wanted an autograph for a niece, and it was a most pleasant affair. There were lots of shiny heads and thick waistlines and even thicker makeup. But there was an acceptance of time, and things gained and lost. People laughed harder and drank less, and no awards were given for meaningless milestones. It was enough that we had come this far. I stayed until the last person left and the night janitors asked me to go home.

On the drive back down the coast I was able to pinpoint the highlight of the evening. It was when Eddy Nunez, one of my closest friends in school, asked me if I still surfed.

"Usually not on the weekends, Eddy, but most other days. Yeah, I'm still hittin' it pretty hard."

The worst part was not getting to speak with Lisa Hecker, to tell her that she had made a difference in my life, to say thanks.

Once you "make it" in professional sports, your experience of it will depend in part on how you define it. When you were a kid, sport was always play; now it's work. As a professional athlete, in the eyes of those who gave you this highly coveted job, you're not a kid who gets paid to have fun playing really well, or moving really fast. You're an entertainer, a commodity, part of the inventory of what makes up the business of sport. But you don't want to think that way. It's too crass, too harsh. Thinking that way won't let you unleash the love of the game that lets you play it so well, that lets you jump over a bar seven feet off the ground or spin four times in the air and land the razor blades strapped to your feet on glassy ice. No, you're no piece of meat, you're a great athlete, god dammit. That's what you are.

And you drink in the moments that remind you of that every day, especially the pure, timeless ones. You swallow those immutably honest moments of athleticism because you know that someday, somehow, you will need the power of ruminative memory. These are a few of my pure moments:

I remember finishing one of my first Ironman races in Kona and looking down to see that my white shoes were now red. I thought,

Didn't I have white shoes? But then I remembered it was blood from the blisters. And I remember the medical director Bob Laird sitting me down, taking off my shoes, and cleaning up those blisters. I remember a local Hawaiian named Curt Tyler walking over and giving me his brand-new sandals right off his feet so that I could walk to my hotel over the hot asphalt. Someone told me he was the mayor of the town.

I remember not believing it when I was actually in the lead of a major race for the first time, until I slowed down and let the sound of my own breath enter the picture. It became a kind of soundtrack to the movie I was watching, only I was also starring in the movie; I was living two lives at the same time, one real and one make-believe, but I couldn't tell the difference until I let all my senses join in the battle.

I remember going to the bank and depositing a prize money check for something like $10,000 and thinking that I had lived a full and rewarding life in college on half of that for an entire year. I told myself not to get used to it. But I think I went out and bought a new guitar that afternoon. It sounded just the same as my old one. And I wondered what had changed.

I know a lot of people who occupy themselves with activities they mostly consider unimportant. Yet those who consider sport relatively unimportant compared to family, health, learning, religion, or economy fail to realize that sport brings us into relationships with all of those important elements of life. That makes it very important. I had developed a true relationship with sport. Sport had become a large part of my social fabric, and I would wear it until it wore out.

Part Two

▼ ▼ ▼ ▼

WAITING FOR THE FILM AT ELEVEN

Heroes: Who Are They Really?

"Maybe we elevate athletes to hero status because, *not in spite of, the fact that they have no real utilitarian value, no real purpose other than some higher meaning to us that we don't fully understand."*

—Anonymous

I don't own much sports memorabilia. Most of the things I procured over my years as a professional have been given away, lost, or dropped into that black hole where lost things go. I do have the original issue of *Surfer Magazine*—or rather my son does, a present to him on the day he was born—and a baseball autographed by the great Los Angeles Dodgers pitcher Sandy Koufax.

I found it the other day, just rolling around the bottom on an empty drawer, banging against the wooden sides. I admired Koufax when I was a kid, still do I guess, and I wondered why. I've never had any real heroes who were public figures, and given the changing face of professional sports, I doubt I will add any athlete heroes anytime soon.

It seems I'm not alone. A poll done in 2001 found that more than half of the people interviewed could not name a public figure whom they considered a hero. Nearly 25% had crossed a name off their hero list for unethical behavior, and one in six had no hero at all. Among those who did, Michael Jordan was the only athlete listed in the top ten, at number nine. Of the remainder, six were dead and three were spiritual leaders.

Since Watergate, Vietnam, and recent revelations of rampant corporate greed from such former stars as Enron, Tyco, WorldCom, and

Adelphia, politicians, war heroes, and captains of industry have not made it easily onto our hero lists. And then there is our ambivalence about creating athlete heroes. Do they fit the established definition of what heroes are, the definition refined over the ages by those who have studied the hero through time: People who distinguish themselves by performing *extraordinary, brave, or noble acts, selflessly*?

It seems that in many ways we are confusing celebrities with heroes, equating fame or achievement with heroic ideals. People are famous for being famous. I'm sure that Vanna White and Kato Kaelin, O.J. Simpson's tenant, are fine people. But what made them recognizable was exposure, not gallantry. The media, in part, has purposely created heroes to hold our attention while the commercials sell us the advertisers' products. Notice that roughly one half of all Olympic television programming shows the athletes not competing but in dramatic exposés—the Up Close and Personal approach. We see a lot of talking heads in preparation for the event, backgrounded by the steady drone of overconfident made-for-TV rhetoric, and not enough of what happens between the starting gun and the finish line.

This constant intrusion, welcome or not, makes it more difficult for the athlete to become a role model, let alone some type of hero. The athletes are demystified just when we want them to compensate for *our* lack of qualities by their actions and behavior. As we project onto them what we aspire to, their every move is camera-chronicled in an effort to expose their feet of clay. We want our heroes to be good, but not godlike. We have to connect to them, and they to us. People relate to the cyclist Lance Armstrong not so much because he is the greatest American cyclist ever, but because he beat an enemy that many of us can relate to—cancer. For the average citizen, the Tour de France is the vaguely recognizable title of "some biking deal over in Europe." Everybody knows somebody who has had cancer.

But what secures Armstrong's inclusion in the category of hero is what he has *done* with his victory over the testicular cancer that nearly killed him. Just as Christopher Reeve dedicated himself to increasing funding for spinal cord research, Lance has gone on the offensive, going after the beast by raising awareness, raising money, and raising the hopes of thousands who look at Lance, see what he has accomplished in sport, and say to themselves, "If Lance can win the Tour de France after surviving cancer, I too will beat it and return to my family, my job, and a normal life."

I have a good friend from Kentucky, a regular school teacher by the name of Mike Caudill who lives on a regular street called Possum Kingdom Road, the operative word being *lives*. You see, if Mike Caudill was truly regular, he would be dead at the hands of leukemia, one more victim with a beautiful wife and a couple of great kids remembering their dad on his birthday and on Christmas and on anniversaries for the rest of their lives. But he's not dead.

I hate cancer. I hate it more than anything else on this earth. I fucking hate cancer because it took my dad away from us. But it also introduced me to Mike Caudill.

It was one of those calls out of the blue. "You don't know me but I have a triathlete friend who has your poster up in his garage and he has cancer now and may need a bone marrow transplant and would you be so kind as to drop him a note of encouragement?"

"Hell yeah." I said. "What's his number and who else does he look up to?"

I hadn't talked to Lance in a year. When I first met him, he was a brash fourteen-year-old; now he was famous. He had won the Tour. He was on TV. He was not easy to reach. But I got to him.

"Lance, there's this fan of yours, a guy named Caudill; seems like a really special guy, you know, one of the types that has a chance. He's a fighter like you, Lance."

Ten minutes later, Lance called Mike Caudill's room in a Kentucky hospital, where he was in thirty days of isolation undergoing bone marrow transplant. Lance was calling between races from a pay phone in Belgium. Mike, drugged and delirious, stared in disbelief at the speakerphone he was unable to reach, half-believing the words he heard were issuing from the poster of Lance Armstrong that was tacked to the wall.

"Hey Mikey, I heard you're having a little problem. Just calling to say you can beat it. Get your ass well and back out there. See you on the road."

Heaven knows we need heroes like Lance because it trickles down. Mike Caudill has become a hero in his own right: Hundreds of kids from his school district will whisper as he walks the hallways, "That's Mr. Caudill. He had an incurable disease and now he's, like, the principal of the whole school. And he's really cool, just a regular guy."

Some athletes play the role of hero well. Some don't even have to act—they earn it off the field with their selfless activities. Others are better at playing the anti-hero—you love to hate him but you never change the channel when he's playing. But the only way to truly guarantee hero status, to play the role perfectly, is to die while you're on top. Jimi and Janis, JFK and Lou Gehrig, James Dean, and Steve Prefontaine—they pulled it off. Dead heroes can't screw up. We'll never see their feet of clay or watch them miss a chord change or an easy fly ball or grow hair in their ears. The only thing that grows is the legend.

I was none of these—not a real hero, not a good actor, not an image-laden star with a gun in the glove compartment. I wasn't even the graceful champion (and I had no Kurt Cobain tendencies lying in wait). I was given just enough to know what it felt like; I was taken backstage for a glimpse of the star's life, but then ushered back to the regular seats. I liked what I'd seen back there—heck, I was normal. But I knew it was thin and unreal and I wouldn't be good at it anyway.

One time I stepped off the stage after delivering a rather short and uninspiring victory speech and was approached by the race director.

"You're weird Tinley," he laughed. "I know you're not cocky but you can easily come across as an unappreciative jerk."

I was kind of stunned. I hadn't said anything boastful.

"What do you mean?"

"I don't know, exactly. It's like you react better to a barb than a compliment."

Many years later I would begin to understand why this man and others had gotten the wrong impression. It's hard to be a champion: to win races, to talk about your race gracefully and honestly, to take pride in your accomplishment—but not too much. I was never very good at it. I always felt uncomfortable in the spotlight but I still sought the tangible benefits that come with success.

In generations past, a hero and his or her myth had time to develop, to simmer and build, before earning their way into our memories and conversations. Not so anymore. It is no wonder we have little loyalty for many athlete stars, and they have little for us. They know the game: It's about entertainment and money. They say, You're only as good as your last home run. Sadly the cliché has the ring of truth.

All this said, the athlete-hero survives and does all those things that heroes are supposed to do: gladden our hearts, ennoble our souls, and show us the vast human potential. Those athlete heroes often earn their status off the field, *performing extraordinary, brave, or noble acts, selflessly*. The great ball player Roberto Clemente is heroic for dying in a plane crash on the way to his earthquake-ravaged homeland of Nicaragua; Cal Ripken, Jr. for his work in creating new opportunities in youth baseball; Magic Johnson for his efforts to increase business opportunities in low-income areas. For them the mantle of heroism is well earned.

Some say that heroes are genetically chosen and must decide whether to embrace their calling. Others argue that the opportunity for heroic deeds exists on every street corner, every day. I think both are right.

Nothing has altered our ideas of heroism like the events of September 11, 2001. Heroes often emerge out of a single, crucial challenge. That tragedy caused us to contrast the nobility of firefighters saving lives in the course of their everyday jobs with, say, Jordan hitting a three-pointer in the NBA finals. Both are great achievements. The difference is in the intent.

The difference, too, is that famous athletes come to believe what they read about themselves. Even the most humble are affected. Every one of us has an ego, which needs a certain amount of love, affection, and admiration. This pretty much keeps us all in the hunt. You cannot wake up every day to the media, your family, your friends, and the public all telling you how great you are and remain unaffected. And then one day you wake up and nobody calls you a hero anymore. And you wonder why not. You wonder if you ever really were.

One of the most talented athletes I know is also one of the most down-to-earth people you could ever meet. He's a surfer, a professional surfer, which is practically an oxymoron. He surfs for a living—a good one—and gets paid to travel around the world. He gets his picture in the surf magazines and rides the best waves. His name is Rob Machado. And yes, he and his surf star buddies have a CD out too.

Like many of the more approachable athletes who have somehow kept their heads out of the clouds, he cites his parents and family for keeping him grounded.

"This one year I won the Ocean Pacific junior title," Rob remembers. "I was sixteen or seventeen and I just walked up the beach and there was, like 20,000 people, you know, and I had just won the OP Junior. I was up on the stage with the trophy, the whole deal. And later we were driving down the Pacific Coast Highway on our way home and pulled up to a stoplight. I was just sitting in the front seat, just like…alrighhhhht, you know? Cool, just feeling all that high of winning. Then this car pulled up next to us…Well, I just looked at them, and my dad looked over at me and he says, 'You think that those people care that you just won the OP Junior?' Just like that he took me off my pedestal, but not in a bad way, it was just like, 'Hey, are you running out? Or you gonna stay on earth with the rest of us?'"

Rob Machado was lucky to have a father like that, a father who cared, a father who knew how to keep his kid grounded, but also how to let him soar.

Yeah, Rob was lucky, as was five-time Olympic gold medal winner Eric Heiden, as was Cal Ripken, Jr., as was John Elway, as was America's greatest miler Steve Scott, and baseball infielder Tim Flannery. The father-son connection in sport is immutable.

If you're a young man and you finally make it to the big leagues, the Olympics, the nationals, or whatever level defines success for you, and your father had a strong hand in getting you there, he is the face you search for in that big crowd, the one you will call a hero.

Everybody thinks that you are the hero; you scored the touchdown, not your dad. And then one day your father is gone and you retire and that golden fame of false heroism turns to ashes. Then the hero must go to that place where heroes have to go, that netherworld of the return. If you ever get the chance, ask John Elway if he would trade his Super Bowl rings to see his dad puttering around the backyard again, to watch him wrestle with his grandkids on the living room floor. I tried for a year to ask him that question. But I already know the answer. I think Elway would trade all of football to have his dad back. I would do the same with my athletic career, all of it for a couple of days out surfing with my dad, my kids sitting on the inside picking off the smaller waves. I'd do it in a minute. And it would last a lifetime.

I remember the first time a kid asked me for an autograph. It was late in the summer of 1982 at the very first major triathlon held in Europe, on the Promenade des Anglais along the Mediterranean Sea near Nice, France. NBC or CBS, I don't remember, was there to film the event, and there were as many camera crews and producer types and French officials in navy blue blazers as there were athletes. I was standing next to my bike in the cool, fog-shrouded morning pumping up my tires when a kid, he couldn't have been more than ten, came up and shoved a little notebook in my face. He addressed me in French, but I could tell by the way his voice ended on a higher note that he wanted something. And his eyes, his little eyes, held a combination of interest, desire, and something else that made me feel uncomfortable, knowing that I could never feed those eyes they way they should be fed.

I glanced around to see if maybe it was a joke; maybe one of my competitors had put the kid up to it. I wasn't famous. Triathlon wasn't soccer or tennis or American basketball. But he didn't know the difference. The kid saw cameras and fast racing bikes and flashy outfits and people deferring to us. The American with the blond hair might be somebody. An autograph signaled that he had gotten close to celebrity, closer to whatever power he imagined I possessed. And further away from what might have been a dull day-to-day life.

I took the little notepad and wrote *bon chance*, good luck, the only French I knew. As an afterthought I scribbled in English "and do your homework." Then I signed my name with a little more flair than I did on checks and speeding tickets.

Imagine playing under the lights on a beautifully manicured field of dreams. Your name is called over the public address speakers and you sprint out to the throbbing sound of 50,000 approving voices. The clamor hits your ears, spreads like wildfire to your brain, and then seeps into your heart. It's a drug, this din, this sign, this language of the masses that says to you, "I love you. You are a hero to me." And you become addicted to this blessed validation of body and soul. At night you sleep the sleep of the adorned. In the morning, you scan the sports pages for your name.

If you're smart or lucky, you will figure this out or someone will explain it all to you. Or maybe, something will happen to put you in that place where you must decide to accept the mantle of hero and the responsibilities that go with it.

Or decline them and maintain the safety of a distant celebrity. Let people buy you drinks. Play golf as "America's Guest."

But to board a plane and fly into the hellish nightmare of several thousand dead from a massive earthquake, thinking that maybe you could grab a shovel and make a difference, well, that is distinguishing oneself in a brave or noble act. It's much harder to pull crumbled concrete and rebar from the wreckage than hit seventy home runs in a season.

Dave Scott, six-time winner of the Ironman Triathlon, was always a great champion. He had a certain presence about him after he won a big race, moving gracefully from group to group, pressing hands and signing autographs with the patience of a parish priest.

I knew Dave well and always wondered how he could project this aura after a long, hard day of racing. I could handle an hour or so and then I would have to excuse myself and slip out the back door and return to the reality that I knew existed just over the hill, just across that fine line between Sunday afternoon and Monday morning.

"Sometimes after an appearance or an event," Dave would say, "I felt like collapsing. The public or the media had painted a picture that was just too overwhelming, too grandiose, that I couldn't live up to the standard. Or maybe it was just me—I've always felt the need to be *on*."

Whether he did his part in the professional athlete paradigm by playing the game well or whether he acted out of an innate sense of responsibility to those who admired him, Dave was always the graceful victor. It didn't make him a hero, but it put him closer than those who shirked their duty to the fans who had lofted them to the hallowed place, if only for a while.

Recently I saw a picture of myself at an awards ceremony at a major championship, one of the last big events where I had done well. Placed in order on the big stage were the top ten men. Some of the men looked tired, most looked satisfied, a few seemed very happy, and one or two were elated.

When I looked at my face, my eyes were flat and deep, like a high mountain lake. They were private, unsharing eyes. They seemed like black open wounds, not angry, not dead, but without life, without the sparkle of direction and purpose. I seemed to be looking past the present and into the dimness of a faraway future that held something other than what I was or what I had achieved.

They weren't hero eyes, not even champion eyes. But eyes that sought. Lonely eyes.

When I saw that picture I tried to recall if I had ever felt like a champion in the twenty-five years I competed. Had I ever earned the right to be standing on a stage for heroic reasons, or were my accolades based only on achieving and retaining a skill that others sought?

After a while I decided that I had made a difference once or twice, but only when I stepped out of my own quest and aligned myself with the dreams of others. The time I stopped during the bike portion of a race to help a competitor change a flat, the time I stayed behind to help the race director pick up trash after the awards ceremony had ended and everybody had gone home. If I ever did any good, it had nothing to do with winning a race.

Truth and Consequences from the Cheap Seats

"It is immaterial whether Magic Johnson will still be able to play basketball at age forty-six. The question is: Can someone who is being paid a million dollars a year for twenty-five years to throw a ball in a basket be tolerated when he misses the basket?"
                                    —John Underwood, *Spoiled Sport*

On May 7, 2003, only a few weeks after Michael Jordan played his last game as a professional athlete, he was cut from a team. The Washington Wizards, the team Jordan had played for his final season, became the first team since Jordan was in the ninth grade to toss out a man considered by most experts to be the best basketball player ever. Jordan had expected to return as team president, the position he held before coming out of retirement to play in two last seasons with the team. But he was not given the chance to transfer his skills to the mental and cerebral side of the court; somebody wasn't confident that his control of the boards would transfer to control of the boardroom. And so Michael Jordan, a man who had made many others in the sporting world millions of dollars, was let go. His Airness was fired.

A large portion of the public, if asked about the lives of professional athletes after they retire, will look at you oddly, as if to say, Why should I even care? They'll say things like, "Why should I give a damn about John Elway? He has enough money to do or be whatever, whoever he wants." Or, "Yeah, these guys were good, but most of them never really leave the sport. They still make money as coaches and TV commentators. Fun jobs, not like working in an office."

There are those who will say that that Darryl Strawberry wasted a huge God-given gift, that he could have been one of the truly great baseball players of all time. The non-empathetic or myopic might go so far as to say that Ali *deserved* Parkinson's disease for fighting Leon Spinks for the world heavyweight title when he was thirty-six years old.

A large percentage of the population could not care less if Bjorn Borg lost most of his vast tennis earnings because of bad business decisions. They look upon pitching great Jim Palmer's comeback try at age forty-five as an attempt to sell more underwear. And that is their choice, their democratic right to judge.

But the truth is they should care. Because the fan's interest in and admiration for the athlete is part of a complex relationship in which both are invested. And, perhaps more importantly, the retiring athlete's heavily compressed life transition can be a model for all those changes that many of us have to face in life. The soldier returning from war, the mother watching her last child leave the house, and the factory worker laid off after thirty years on the job all experience sudden and dramatic changes in life that are a shock to the order of their existence.

Dramatic change is never easy. They don't teach you how to get fired, get divorced, or face a chronically sore back in school. People should care, because no matter how envious we may be of an athlete's lifestyle or all the money he may or may not have earned, emotional trauma deserves compassion. If retired athletes go on to become politicians and captains of industry, the public helped put them there. If they die under a bridge, homeless, hungry, and forgotten, we put them there too.

When you're an athlete, the public is ready, willing, and able to offer adulation and with it immediate and intense gratification. And when you're done, well, you had better appreciate all the good times you had as a player, because for many people, "ex-professional athlete" means the same thing as ex-anything—you're done.

Cynicism about retiring athletes and their troubles is nothing new. Roman gladiators entertained the masses and were returned to slavery if they hadn't earned their freedom in the coliseum. Jim Thorpe, arguably one of the greatest athletes of all time, died a penniless alcoholic in 1953. Few people seemed to care back then. After all, they said, he was part American Indian, and he shouldn't have been drinking.

When the great NBA center Wilt Chamberlain died of a heart attack in October of 1999 at the age of sixty-three, much of the press couldn't help but refer to his claim (made in his autobiography, *A View from Above*) of having slept with 20,000 women. They focused on the man's chosen lifestyle first, his contributions to the world of sport second, and then finally his untimely and tragic death.

A businessperson works long and hard to move up the corporate ladder. An academic never stops doing research. Teachers must constantly renew their skills and knowledge of the latest materials. Same for doctors, lawyers, plumbers, and engineers. Men and women work hard to attain "membership" in a community of like-minded professionals and industry workers. And once they've got it, they don't give it up easily.

For an athlete, that syndrome is even more pronounced. Out of approximately one million kids who play football in some organized form, only 40,000 will ever play at the college level. And of those, maybe 1,500 will make it to the NFL. That is a very exclusive community, one that is as tight knit as any professional community on earth. The players work extremely hard to achieve that status. That esprit de corps and camaraderie are nearly irreplaceable. When you are *in* the group, you are truly in. But when you are out, you are way *out*.

And it can all be taken away from you in a fleeting moment: an unfortunate accident, a career-ending injury, some young kid coming up through the ranks who is just a bit faster and a bit stronger than you. Shazam. You're gone. A doctor can be a doctor until the day he or she dies. So strong is the pull to keep playing that the players will *always* play hurt or injured. A lot of people don't understand this. The fans only see the players in the NFL on Sunday. They don't know the pain they put up with Monday through Saturday.

The average NFL player, depending on position, lasts three to five years. And yet, because of the status of football in America, a half a million boys and men will get hurt playing the game in any given year, 45,000 of them requiring some type of operation to repair the injury.

Those numbers don't make the game highlights and they aren't discussed around the water cooler on Monday morning. No, it's more like, "If that Jones hadn't missed that block." The fans don't know that the vast majority of those 40,000 college players never receive an actual degree from a university. They don't know that there are other numbers besides touchdowns and RBIs and triple doubles and career assists.

They might know that Raiders Hall of Fame center Jim Otto played sixteen seasons in the NFL, including a team record of 210 consecutive games. But they don't know that he's had at least thirteen football-related operations, including two shoulder replacements, some thirty concussions, twenty broken noses, a detached retina, a broken jaw, broken ribs, two broken knee caps (one was completely removed), 150 stitches in his face, and countless sprained ankles, sprained wrists, and pulled muscles. They don't know that he wakes up every morning feeling like he's been run over by a truck. They don't know that he was diagnosed with cancer in 2002, or that he still works for the Raiders organization.

"Usually, when someone asks me what I do with the Raiders," he said, "I tell them 'pretty much anything I want to'...I've been there forty-three years. I know the organization."

Fans also might not know that his replacement at center for the Raiders, Dave Dalby, felt constant pressure to play injured during his long tenure in the league. Or that Dalby struggled in life after football and died in a car accident in 2002 when the van he was driving hit a tree.

The cynics look at pro athletes and see only the fame and the money and the perks. They can say, quite accurately, that the team sport guys really haven't had to make any difficult decisions since high school. The team, or the league, or one of their managers made those choices for them. But they don't realize that this is a curse when the game is finally over and the players have to learn all those things at age twenty-five, thirty, or thirty-five.

"You don't have a season to get ready for anymore," former Raiders coach John Madden once said. "You don't have a game to get ready for. You don't have to go lay it on the line. So you don't get ready for anything."

Sports fans don't hear a great deal about athletes who founder after retiring. Too much would be bad for TV ratings. After a particularly brutal sack of the quarterback, the fans are not reminded that virtually all long-term players in the NFL will suffer from some form of spinal compression. As the cameras pan across the home team's bench, showing a player patting another player on the back as he comes off the field, the expert commentator won't tell the viewing audience that many athletes report feeling "abandoned" upon retirement, as some athletes report. Or that they "feel like a lost kid," that their spouses wondered aloud too many times what happened to the big, strong hero they married.

Indeed, it's easy to be crass about professional athletes, especially the ones who are crass with the fans who buy the tickets that pay for their huge salaries. But even if much of the fans' cynicism is earned by a player's antisocial off-court behavior, we still must look beneath the problems and begin to study and understand the inherent difficulties in every major transition in life.

Three years after I had retired, I woke up one morning with a sore back and a desk full of bills, which I was wondering how I could pay without dipping into our retirement savings again. Worst of all, when I looked in the mirror, my hair looked darker than I remembered it being since I was a kid. Granted this seems vain, but bear with me. Sun-bleached hair had always been a marker, a measuring stick, the outward sign that I was living the life I wanted to live—outside, in the sun. I wished right then that time had halted fifteen years ago at the apex of my blond innocence. Most of my older friends had lost a lot of their hair, and what they kept had returned to its natural color as a life of sailing, surfing, and biking under the California sun was traded for a career under the fluorescent bulbs of offices and warehouses. And everything they stood for.

I looked in the mirror and realized for the first time that I was nearing middle age. I was no longer a young, immortal, pro jock. I was in my early forties, somewhere between life's front and back nine. And it scared the shit out of me. Then the phone rang. It was my friend David Bailey.

When Bailey calls you, something profound usually happens. Because David Bailey, former national motocross champion, husband, father, artist, TV commentator, paraplegic, winner of the Ironman Triathlon in the hand-crank cycle/wheelchair division, never calls anyone back.

"Whatta ya doing Tinley?"

"Writing."

"No you're not."

"Okay, so I just realized that I'm gonna die one day."

"That's cool. What took you so long?"

"My hair had to turn brown again."

"So dye it."

"Gimme a break. That's not the point. Besides, you know I won't even buy pre-faded jeans."

"At least you could if you weren't such a damn purist."

"What's your point Bailey?"

"Your blond fades to brown. My legs fade to twigs in this chair. You realize you're not fuckin' Peter Pan. I realize I might not walk in my lifetime. Hey Tinley…"

"Yeah Dave?"

"Keep me out of your book. I don't want anybody feeling sorry for me."

Joe Namath was one of the most popular quarterbacks in the history of the NFL. His virtual guarantee of a New York Jets Super Bowl victory in 1969 is the stuff of legend. At sixty years old he is in pain, all the time. Namath has had two knee replacements since his retirement in 1977. He also has pain in his thumbs and left hip. "I haven't had a solid night's sleep since I can remember," he said. But Namath says this matter-of-factly, not with self-pity in his voice; he's just reporting, not complaining. He knows that he won't get much sympathy.

▼ ▼ ▼

Many of the early players in the league couldn't earn enough to support themselves on football alone. Don Maynard, Namath's teammate on the 1969 Super Bowl-winning Jets, held another job in the off-season after he started in 1958. The average salary in the NFL in the 1950s was $15,000. It didn't reach $100,000 until 1982—a lot of money still, but not nearly the $735,000 it was in 2002.

Some of these guys don't want any pity. All they want is respect. Sammy Winder, an NFL player for nine seasons, including three Super Bowl appearances with the Denver Broncos, never made more than $400,000. Even in today's dollars, that's some good coin.

"You have to go on," Winder told the *San Diego Union-Tribune*. "You don't have a choice. You go to a normal life or go sleep under a bridge." Of course, it can also be said that if you made $400,000 for several years in a row and invested it prudently, you could buy a few bridges.

The years when the money's coming in are no problem. It's the years that follow, when you're finished doing what you felt you were born to do. Then money can be a curse if you have it, because you don't *have* to do anything. Of course, it's a curse when you ain't got it either.

Probably the most disturbing statistic of all about the NFL is reported by Bob Glauber of *Newsday*: "Since 1980, seven former players have committed suicide, five of them since 1987. In addition, one player committed suicide while still on an NFL roster. There have been five suicides combined among players of the three other major sports since 1980. The suicide rate among former NFL players is nearly six times the national average of 12.1 per 100,000 population." No money, no respect, no future—no life.

Sport has changed in recent years. And many of those changes have to do with the pressure to produce events that will play well on television. Outdoor motocross races were virtually unheard-of in the U.S. until the concept of arena-based Super-Cross hit the market, and these high-flying, high-crashing daredevils were made into seven-figure household names. Or they ended up in a wheelchair, like David

Bailey. In triathlon, never considered a spectator sport, the very nature of the sport as an individual endurance event was altered with
the advent of legalized drafting on the bicycle portion. For more exciting, TV-friendly racing, we were told. Most major league baseball
players will swear that the ball is wound tighter these days, making it
harder, livelier, and easier to hit out of the ballpark. Why? Because
baseball's popularity was on the wane and the fans love to see home
runs. The league of course denies this.

NBA officiating sure seems lax these days. When I grew up, basketball wasn't considered the contact sport it is today. And hockey?
Well, we've all heard the joke about going to a fight and seeing a
hockey game break out.

I remember being at the start of one event in the Survival of the
Fittest competition. It was a very challenging run over Volkswagen-
sized rocks, through rivers they referred to as streams, across a botan-
ical garden of surfaces. The organizers lined us up, told us to follow
the flags on the edge of the course, and fired the starting gun.

I had gotten a good start, as I was anxious to do well. Thirty seconds later I heard a whistle and all the competitors were called back.
What was the problem? Alligators spotted in the stream? A lightning
storm moving in? No. They wanted another camera angle for the
start. We'd have to restage it. Welcome to made-for-TV sports. "It's
worth it guys," they told us. "Wait 'till you see the show."

The most far-reaching change in the Big Four sports of America,
though, has to be in the size of the average NFL offensive lineman.
They just keep getting bigger and bigger and bigger, as do the consequences for the men who play both sides of the line.

In 1975 there wasn't a single lineman over 300 pounds. By 1990
there were 39; in 2002 there were 327. What happened? The rules were
changed. In 1978 the NFL changed its fundamental blocking rule.
Before then, offensive linemen were not allowed to extend their arms
and lock their elbows. The better linemen were lighter and quicker, no
different than the defensive line. But with the advent of the new rule,
the emphasis went from agility and mobility to another kind of
Sunday mass.

The situation now breeds a high risk of heart disease and muscle-tendon-ligament damage in nearly every player who bulks up beyond what his body is designed to be. In 1994, the National Institute for Occupational Safety and Health (NIOSH) conducted a mortality study at the request of the NFL Players Association, which was concerned about reports that retired NFL players were dying at a higher rate than the average American. The study, which included 6,848 players from 1959 to 1988, actually found the opposite to be true—except in the case of lineman. NIOSH reported that offensive and defensive linemen had a 52% greater risk of dying of heart disease than the general population.

Now, it would be easy to slough this whole thing off with a "well, it's their decision" kind of attitude. But remember that where the pros go, college players, and ultimately high school players, may follow.

And there is always that nagging question of why. Why did the league change the rules? With more players than ever getting hurt and retiring with disabling injuries, and no end in sight for the growth of some of these players, why not change it back, effectively reversing the trend? Sure, and roll back the price of gas while you're at it.

"It's all about the offensive scoring," said one retired player who requested anonymity. "It's about making the game more fan-friendly with lots of time for the QB to find his receivers. Man, the fans have to see touchdowns to be happy."

If we are to believe this line of thinking (and this anecdote was well supported in numerous interviews with NFL players, both retired and active), then it is not a stretch to make the connection between ancient Rome and modern day football.

"The whole thing has 'gladiatorialized' the players," my source continued. "If you end up on the bottom of a pile of players on the line and the average weight is 280 instead of 230, that's a big difference in how you feel when you get up...if you get up."

But nobody ever thinks about that: not the starry-eyed kid watching the game on TV with his dad, not the guy on top of the pile. That's just football, they say, that's the way the game is played.

Or is it? I called David Bailey back. I wanted to apologize for freaking out about my hair. It was just a momentary slip; some mental fog had blanketed my common sense. I wanted to tell him I could lift this velvet noose from around my neck and accept the natural order of things. I didn't care if my back was sore, I'd stretch it. I didn't care if I wasn't rich anymore, we'd downsize. I wanted to tell him I didn't give a flying fuck whether people respected what I had done or not. I couldn't control them any more than I could pick the hour and the minute of my last breath. I wanted to tell my friend David Bailey because he had made the decision to live, regardless of whether he had to chase his kids around the block by pushing himself in a chair. As I waited for the someone to pick up the phone, I heard a dog barking in the background and the sound of a jukebox being turned up somewhere down the block. Something had momentarily degraded my spirit and I had lost grace in my words to a friend who didn't need to witness my petty inner battles. I'd fix it with Dave, probably learn something too.

But I couldn't. His wife answered the phone. Dave wasn't there anymore. He had gone to the pool to swim. "But he'll call you back."

Time and Space:
Records and the Long Run

"The seven gold medals count, of course, but what is more important to me is that I did the best I could, and when I finished I was on top."
— Mark Spitz, Olympic gold medal winner

thletes who hold records, however briefly, control time, simply for having done something faster, higher, longer, or farther than any other man or woman. Those whose names are listed in the record books are top dog, for the moment. They are the kings and queens for the day.

But their reign is usually short-lived. In Olympic swimming competition, for instance, it is quite common for a competitor to hold the world record for a day, maybe two, between the qualifying heats and the finals. That's hardly enough time to e-mail your sponsors to invoke the contract clause that awards you a bonus for such a feat.

Other records take years and years to compile. It took Cal Ripken, Jr. sixteen years to play his 2,632 consecutive games. Wayne Gretzky's 2,857 points and Henry Aaron's 755 home runs both required an entire career. These are the numbers the fans remember and revere the most because they grow up with them, counting them like months and years, birthdays and anniversaries of their own lives. The athletes seem immortal.

Records of space are only slightly different from records of time. They remind us how large our universe is, and how very small. They become part of our vernacular. Home runs don't just go out of

the ballpark; they go into the *upper deck, out of the park, all the way to
the moon.*

We continue to marvel not only at how fast a man or woman can
run, but how far. We are more taken by the long drive in golf than by
the finesse required to win. *Drive for show, putt for dough.*

Nearly all of the world's tallest mountains have been scaled.
Hundreds of cyclists endeavor each year to *qualify* for the right to
enter the Race Across America, a nonstop 3,000-mile epic. The
Hawaiian Ironman is now considered a medium-distance event because it only takes a day to finish—the winners cross the line with
their sunglasses on to prove they made it before dark.

And what about the Whitbread Round the World yacht race? Is
that long enough? Or should the sailors turn around and come back
the other way?

There is something mystically attractive about numbers and distances in sport. They ground us in a world that is trying its damnedest
to disconnect us from ourselves. Still I can't help but wonder if some
of the awe in sport has been compromised by the unceasing effort to
sell and market and hype that part of the human spirit that creates
these feats, the place where talent and desire, art and muscle, intangi-
bly come together. How can we accurately score the grace and beauty
of an ice skater or a gymnast?

It took a while before I fully realized that my corporate sponsors, no
matter how well I got along with them, weren't paying me because I
was a nice guy. I was selling product for them. I suppose I knew this
early on in my career but I chose to ignore it because it was flattering
to be sponsored, to be recognized with a check in the mail every
month. It was one more marker that I was making it on my own terms.

Or was I? My growing idealism about what sport was *supposed* to
be was leaking into my everyday thoughts and actions. When I criti-
cized the actual state of pro sports, my friends called me cynical. My
wife called me ungrateful. They were both right and wrong. And on
the night I was accepted into the Triathlon Hall of Fame, I carried that
inner conflict up to the stage and right into the microphone.

Bill Smith, the father of former triathlon world champion Spencer Smith and a wonderfully tactless man whom I had grown very fond of, could see I was nervous. "Get over here Tinman, you bloody poofter," he bellowed in his thick cockney accent. "Let Uncle Smitty buy you a cocktail before you's getting up there."

It was supposed to be a big night and, yes, I was a little nervous. I wanted to show the appreciation that I felt, my gratitude for all that I had been given. Part of the ceremony was a film showing the highlights of my career. As honored as I was, it still felt a little like I was watching my own funeral. And as I listened to the introduction, the recitation of numbers—victories, years competing, former records—all the empirical evidence that proved I deserved the recognition, I began to wonder why I was being inducted before others who had amassed better numbers, others who'd put up the kind of numbers that don't get your mug on TV. Race directors, medical support staff, volunteers, bike mechanics. Racing was the easy part. Picking up three thousand little squashed Dixie cups from the side of the road every weekend—that was putting up numbers.

My socialist politics had risen to the surface from the bottom of Bill Smith's third shot of tequila. The timing was really, really bad. I got up on stage, slurred a few thanks. I called my wife "a good *ho*" to whom I was indebted, adding coyly that I'd probably keep her around a bit. Then I sat down to an embarrassed silence broken only by the raucous laughter of Bill Smith from the back of the ballroom.

"You show 'em boy. You're in the hall of shame now, matey!"

Smart athletes know it could all end tomorrow. They *should* know, anyway. Even if they fail to admit it—to think about a torn rotator cuff, a snapped femur, one too many concussions—the possibility must be lurking in the back of their mind.

But if they held a record, or were awarded membership in some exclusive group within their sport, the pressure is eased. A record cannot be taken away. It's not immortality, but it's a legacy. The record is perennial, like the grass on the playing field.

Time builds up legacies, it doesn't break them down. There is a story from the short yet appealing history of triathlon that still gets bantered around. It concerns a single workout that my friend and training partner Kenny Souza and I did two weeks before a Hawaiian Ironman in the early 1990s. It started out innocently enough, a series of intervals: eight fast runs of four hundred meters around a local high school track, with two-hundred-meter jogs in between. As the legend goes, the workout ended two hours later after Souza and I had run *fifty* repeats of four hundred meters, all because neither of us wanted to be the one to say, "That's enough, you're the man, I give up." In truth, we ran twenty-five, but that's the point—like a fish story, or a story about being at Woodstock or seeing an apparition of the Virgin Mary, the tale is misrepresented over time, magnified, and the legend becomes truth because we want it to be.

Sometimes I look at my knees and think they resemble a collection of mutated cells viewed under a high school microscope, or pinkish-red ripples on the ocean's surface, a photograph taken at sunset from a helicopter. They've been banged, bruised, scraped, ripped, and de-fleshed. They've been used as bony training wheels, outriggers, and tripods on every form of terra firma from asphalt and Astroturf to rocks, sand, rubble, and reconstituted rip-rap. And triathlon is not ex-actly considered a contact sport.

If nothing else, my knees tell a story. If you sliced through the scar tissue evenly, you might be able to reconstruct my athletic history, like counting the rings of a tree trunk or examining the fossil of some strange prehistoric fish. The insides, however, work like well-oiled sewing machines. And that amazes me. There but for fortune go my knees: topographical maps of gnarled flesh that house the machinery to run twenty miles if the spirit moved me. And if the rest of the ve-hicle were willing and able.

Some days I wake up feeling like someone has walked over my grave, like I have been divided and conquered. Other days, after cof-fee, a hot shower, cold OJ, and a few solitary moments to loosen the bands that hold my body together—I feel pretty darn good. Like, hot damn, I ain't forty-something, bring those lazy young punks on. Reality lies between these extremes. By the time noon rolls around, I've landed somewhere to the left of middle, where the body works just fine, thank you very much, at least within the confines of "regular guy" training. Still I forget what I have asked of my body over twenty years of denial that someday I might actually wake up with a sore back, same as my uncle, my granddad, and the sixty-three-year-old insurance salesman down the road who shakes his finger at me when he sees me running and says, "You oughta pace yerself young man, you'll see"—still I refuse to let age control my advancement in time.

When I went back to graduate school in 1999 all the students looked really young. They would call me sir, thinking I was one of the instructors coming in on his day off dressed in shorts and a T-shirt, with a backpack slung over his shoulder instead of the standard-issue brown leather briefcase. Indeed, it was a bit unnerving at first, trying to fit in, or at least not stand out. I had grown up, god dammit. How did that happen?

The gap didn't last long though. When I found a few older people to hang around with, twenty-eight instead of twenty-two, when I had been assigned my own class to teach, the chasm closed, or at least narrowed to some acceptable width.

I have long understood that it is impossible to stop the hands of time. You can slow them down considerably with a good diet, low stress, cooperative genes, and exercise; but the clock still moves. The old soldiered athlete must accept this sooner or later. He or she must begin to realize that it is okay, as Max Ehrmann writes in *Desiderata*, to "gracefully surrender the things of youth."

No, this isn't easy. For younger athletes who retire before they are ready, maybe not of their own volition, it is especially hard—as hard as it is to understand the Zen concept that we are not moving through time as much as it is moving through us.

You can sit back and look at what you did. Maybe you held a record for a period of time, something decisively non-global. You won fourteen games of handball in a row in sixth grade, or ran the most laps in the high school jog-a-thon until some kid from the south side transferred in; maybe you once did more sit-ups than all the guys in the club, and won the $22 betting pool and the respect of your peers. You hold those numbers in reverence somewhere in your head. These small reminders are pugmarks of your journey as an athlete. That's what I do with my knees: I think, wow, they're chewed up, but even after logging enough miles to get to the moon and not quite back, they sure work good. Those scars give me rights. To what I am not sure, but rights nonetheless.

Possibly it's the right to admit I screwed up, that I wasted time in sport, that I played too long. Possibly it's the right finally to be the good champion, long after anyone would remember that I once was a champion, that I held the world record at the Ironman distance for one year. Or possibly it's the right to slow down and enjoy everything else in life, things that now seem infinitely more important than records or streaks or how far the ball flew. Watching the unmitigated surprise and delight on my wife's face when I bring her home a flower picked on a run; waking up early and feeling that the smell of good, strong coffee will be enough to ensure a good, strong day. Winning close to one hundred races in my career gives me the right to be simple, to be romantic, to reacquaint myself with things I used to dismiss as schmaltz, things I never should have lost. But thank God some of it is coming back.

These are things that round you out a bit, smooth the edges. I wouldn't call my edges smooth yet, but you certainly can't shave your face with them like you used to be able to.

For many people time is an enemy, a thief of all things young, all things new, clean, springy, and guilt-free. But for the aging athlete, and for anybody willing to understand and finally accept the benefits of advancing years, time can be a friend. It comes knocking quietly at first, then a bit louder, like a rainstorm moving up a dry and thirsty valley— a friend bringing gifts of knowledge and wisdom. Even with wet and muddy shoes, you must let him in. For he has much to teach you.

Places They Go

*"We walked through the parking lot. Neither of us said
anything. We thought the world had ended."*
—Anne Ryun, wife of miler Jim Ryun,
speaking about one of Ryan's last races
where he had failed to reach his goal.

You will remember the hotel rooms. Some you will miss and
not know why. Others you won't miss, though you think
you should. So many hotel rooms, rooms filled with ghosts
of the past: events, liaisons, card games, songs written on
guitar heard only by four thin walls papered in a pale yellow daisy
pattern. They're always pale yellow daisies, with matching bed-
spreads that reek of a thousand travel-weary bodies.

Hotel rooms are sanctuaries for the professional athlete. And
prisons. You move from town to town, crowded airport to crowded
airport, thinking only of plopping your travel-weary body down on
the daisy-patterned bed, taking your shoes off, having a shower hot
enough to wipe the day away but not quite burn your thick skin.
You're sick of people in your face all day: fans, umpires, coaches,
sponsors, other players. Most of them are there to help, but they
only want to help in their own way. You recognize that but they
often don't; their efforts are veiled in the glee of closeness to a real
sports hero.

But it's not always just your way. You're the pro? Remember?
Your weariness and ego have blinded you to this fact as well. But the
shower felt good, you're hungry, and you could use a beer. Just one
tall cold one. You pick up the phone and dial the rooms of the people

you were sick of forty minutes ago. Moods and hotel rooms, like the life of a professional athlete, are transient.

Sometimes you leave the door slightly ajar, a signal that visiting athletes, media types, and miscellaneous supporters are welcome, that you're lonely. Come on in. You become each other's mechanics, therapists, confidants, friends, and priests. You become one being, maybe a more balanced person, because you took time to help a competitor, an archrival. You're unique, but you're the same.

I remember staying in a ten-room hotel on the outskirts of Panama City, Panama for a race. A female competitor kept knocking on my door.

"Can I borrow a five-millimeter Allen wrench?'

"What kind of tires do you think I should run tomorrow?"

"Do you think Carol is in good running shape?"

All I could think of was insecurity and obsession, the twin traits of the endurance athlete. They belonged to both of us—her for projecting her fear onto me, and me for allowing it to enter. She was obsessed with details. I was insecure about why I wasn't.

"Bring your fucking bike over and I'll fix it. We'll talk about your race strategy."

"I can't believe you'd do that for me."

Honey, it ain't just for you. I'm just passing some goodwill forward.

Hotel rooms are unlikely spots for your darkest moments and highest highs. At worst they are prisons where you lie awake at night worrying about tomorrow's *big game*, wrestling with the demon of self-doubt until you beat him by beating your own fears and insecurities.

Athletes will tell you that they get their mental strength through mind exercises, sport psychology, and the training itself, all of which is surely true. Still I can't help but believe that steely-eyed courage is often honed on the daisy bedspread of a nameless hotel.

Hotel rooms can also be places of victory celebration, much more so than award ceremonies or locker rooms. You could be sitting around an old, dingy room reeking of smoke and old sex and Dial soap and mothballs, entertainment courtesy of a television that receives two local channels. Or you could be in a three-bedroom suite with a view of the park and champagne chilling in a silver vase. Either way, if the room holds only those who have *earned* the right to feel that victory in the deepest parts of their gut, then the room becomes magical. It is an honor to be with the others, to jump on the beds, throw ice at each other, brag about your own performance, or allow others to lie about theirs. Nobody complains about the noise. Sporting victories are infectious. Other hotel guests are more likely to bring extra ice than pound on the walls and yell for quiet.

Airports are stress factories for the constant traveler. Traveling once was a stimulating way to experience the unique textures and nuances of local culture, a way to connect with people from lands near and far, to appreciate how small our planet really is.

Now, with the advent of high-speed, low-cost mass movement, everybody wants to go somewhere, and not necessarily to experience a foreign city and its people. They just want to pop in, get a quick glimpse of the highlights, and be back at their desks by Monday morning. Airports have become the fast-food eateries of travel.

And professional athletes, by virtue of their need to compete against the best in the world, need airports. I suppose we are lucky to have them. In the days of trains and buses and ships, you would rarely have a chance to train or compete with the best from around the globe.

I can remember sitting in the spa after a really hard swim at the University of California, San Diego, looking around at a dozen men and women, some of the best triathletes in the world, most of them friends. And thinking, oh my gosh, there are nine countries represented in this pool of hot water—a miniature, bubbly United Nations for jocks.

Without airports this would not have been possible. They came to San Diego because the best were there, somehow hoping that some of the magic would wear off on them. They came in airplanes.

One year I logged close to 100,000 miles in the air chasing events, competitors, and prize money from Rio to Sydney to Tokyo to Helsinki to Paris. And that was the early season. The race directors would gladly provide two tickets and accommodations for my wife and me. My daughter Torrie was under two years old and flew for free, so off we went. Everywhere. Torrie would run down the hallways of unnamed hotels in countries that blurred together in that wonderful period of innocence when every room had a view and every race a purpose.

Back then, the flights weren't so crowded and the airports were almost breezy. Terrorism was not the threat that it is now. The odd hijacking in some foreign country didn't seem to bother us. We were young, the money was good, and each new country was another pushpin on the wall map that illustrated my journeys. Traveling and racing: two half circles meeting in the middle to make a whole. Only it was back then and could never happen again. The thought of airports now gives me a sick feeling in the pit of my stomach. It raises my blood pressure. I hate airports.

Near the end of my career, the budget travel revolution in full swing, I began to cope by cutting my in-and-out time. Friends who used to be jealous of my journeys became incredulous.

"Where'd you go this week?"

"Had a race in Nice, France."

"How was the trip, the weather, all the sights?"

"Can't remember, really. Been there eight times before. Same race, same course."

"How'd you do?"

"Fourth, maybe third. Yeah, I think it was third. Made a few grand. It'll make the house payment this month."

"Wow, you were at the run on Tuesday. You must have been gone only five or six days."

"Four. And that was too many. I think I can do it in three next year."

One year I was checking my bike in at the United Airlines counter at Tokyo's Narita Airport. I was on my way back from a disappointing finish at the Japan Ironman and was anxious to get on the long flight, fall asleep, and wake up having forgotten the whole thing. The customer service agent told me my bike was four pounds over the excess baggage limit I had just paid for, and then informed me she would have to charge a freight fee of $300. I took a deep breath and reminded her that I had probably logged a half a million miles on her airline since she had begun logging her own time toward a pension. But rules were rules.

A supervisor, sensing the rising tension, asked if I could possibly take a few things out of my bike case to get it under the limit. I was all too happy to do so, because it would allow me to graphically depict the other side of working in a "service industry." I opened my bike case and spilled across the first-class counter all my sweat-stained laundry, including my blood- and urine-soaked racing shoes and other detritus accumulated over two weeks in hotel rooms smaller than most camper shells. I took out a ten-pound tool kit, reweighed the case, and then in plain view put the tool kit back in the case, closed it up, set it on the scale with my left foot supporting the back edge just a bit...and smiled at them. As we walked away with our boarding passes, my friend looked at me and told me I had balls. No, I told him, I'm just tired of airports.

Another time I did a short race in Chicago. With over five thousand competitors going off in wave-starts of one hundred athletes or so every five minutes, it took almost five hours just to start everybody. The pros went off first and finished in about an hour and forty-five minutes. The slower age-group athletes would take three, even four hours.

I rode my bike back to the hotel, threw it in a box and grabbed a cab for the airport, hoping to make an earlier flight. I arrived just in time with my race numbers still inked on my arms and legs, as I had skipped a shower. I was home sitting at my kitchen table in Del Mar while competitors were still on the course, two thousand miles away. I was proud of that. I had beaten the airports at their own game.

And then there are the quiet places, the places that athletes go to prepare themselves for an event, to put their mind in that unique state that will allow them to put forward all that is available to them. And if they're lucky, more.

The overused image would have them sitting on an old oak bench in front of their locker, staring at the dank, concrete floor, head down as if in deep prayer. They have their uniform on. It is clean and crisp after a fresh wash, although there are stains of a certain kind that can never be removed: reminders of a race run in shoes bloodied by blistered toes, jerseys with grass stains from a diving catch, a gracefully violent tackle; markers that are meant to remain because to erase the blood and earth and sweat is to erase the memory.

This image works. And is a part of nearly every athlete's career at some point. Locker rooms, maybe even more than hotels, are hallowed places for the team player. This is where a group of men or women can become a form of human succession, an athletic lineage, an outgrowth of all the work and preparation they have invested in their job. And all that those before and after will have invested.

Or locker rooms can be moldy hellholes of discontent when the unit falls into disarray; a place where nobody wants to be, at a time when no one wants to be with each other. Lonely. Smelly. Dark. It could have been something else altogether—if they'd won. But the genealogy continues nonetheless, in darkness and in bright sunshine.

We all find our own locker rooms to prepare ourselves. The place is part of the ritual of preparation. My races were always early, often at 7:00 A.M.: early enough to close the roads to traffic but just light enough for the athletes to see. My wake-up call was at 4:20 A.M., regardless of whether the race started at 6:30, 8:00, or even 9:00. It was a number that I started using early in my career, a number that was also the title of my favorite song by my favorite rock group, "4+20" by Crosby, Stills, and Nash.

I loved that song. But there was nothing I hated more in my career than hearing the alarm on race day, looking at the clock, and seeing those numbers: 4:20 A.M.

Once I was up and going it got easier, the butterflies releasing slowly as I put myself in that special place, readying my body and mind for the task of the day, for the pain of high-level, high-stakes competition.

Now, in nearly every region of the world north of 30°N latitude, it is dark at 4:20 A.M. during the summer months. I needed to move, though, to wake my body up, warm up the muscles, push the blood through its own darkened streets: *burning the tires,* I called it.

So by 4:45 A.M. I was out on the dark streets of some city in some country, sometimes lost, running, burning my tires.

That was my place, those predawn streets; that was my locker room. And I saw much: destitute homeless men lying in gutters in Rio and Manhattan, early-morning delivery boys on bikes with baskets full of bread in the south of France, late-night partygoers leaving the nightclub district of Munich, and farmers wearing heavy, sheepskin-lined coats climbing into old lorries near Christchurch, New Zealand.

They are images rich in texture, deeply imbedded in my memory. But they also carry with them a heavy sense of loneliness. I was an athlete; my playing field took me all over the world. I *belonged* on the road a certain period of every year.

In the beginning the travel was alluring, seductive. Then it got lonely. Near the end of my career, the trips got shorter in time and distance. The last year I competed as a pro, I flew to only three races, and that was because they paid me to show up and it was too far to drive.

I needed the stability of home, my own bed, my family and friends; it's the same for anybody who is away for extended periods. For an individual starting a new career and, in many ways, a new life, the concept of home becomes crucial. It is not just a physical location, but a sense of security when so many other aspects of one's life seem insecure. Home is a launching platform, a fallback position, a safe house, a haven. Home is a place you can return to when you succeed and when you fail and be treated the same. When an athlete retires, he or she needs a good home.

But sometimes athletes have been on the road for so long they have lost contact with any single geographical location; they don't have a real home. The road was their home, the team and the other competitors their family. These athletes have to find a spot, a place that serves that purpose.

Some evidence, mostly anecdotal, indicates that a large percentage of retired athletes resettle in small towns. Maybe they dislike the inherent duplicity of the big city. Maybe they need to feel like big fish, if only in a small pond. And maybe it's just quiet and peaceful and they can afford to work part-time, traveling to the city if need be. In any case, I have that desire. And I've heard many athletes speak of settling down in little beach or mountain towns and finding that sense of community they once had in their sport, that sense of connection that was lost when it all ended.

The great American Olympic skier Billy Kidd did just that: He found a town, found what he calls "the best job in the world," and could not be happier about it.

Steamboat Springs, Colorado, has produced more Olympians per capita than any city in America. If you are an alpine skier, a Nordic skier, a Nordic Combined skier (Nordic skiing and ski jumping), or a ski jumper, there is a good chance you would consider Steamboat as a home.

Billy Kidd's job title is "Director of Skiing." He does marketing and promotions for the mountain, but his true value is in his accessibility to people, his love of skiing, and his love of skiers. Almost every day he skis with visitors on the mountain, showing them around, offering tips, being a host. The man gets paid to ski for fun. And he dreads the day he can't go to work. That's a place we all aspire to, regardless of who we are and what we do.

I was there one winter to ski for a few days. Reaching into my wallet to pull out a credit card to pay for a lift ticket, I noticed another card that had come in the mail around Christmas from somebody in their marketing department, a girl I had met at a mountain bike race the summer before. As an afterthought, I handed the little piece of plastic to the cashier and asked if it might give me a small discount.

"Mr. Tinley, this is a season pass. How many days would you like at the moment?" I would remember these people and this place.

When We Were Kings

"Today, I consider myself the luckiest man in the world."
—Lou Gehrig, New York Yankee and
Hall of Famer, as he retired

Jimmy and I were sitting out on a wide, verdant strip of grass overlooking the ocean. It was Maui. It was sunset. The tropical air floated around us like a birthday cloud surrounds a three-year-old. We had a cooler full of frosties. And we were playing guitars.

The morning's race had gone well for both of us. The season was over. We were in Hawaii. Drinking beer. Playing old Buffett tunes.

"You reckon it gets any better?"

"Don't see how."

"Think it's all been worth it?"

No answer.

"How much longer you reckon you'll race?"

No answer. A key change into a new song. Seamless. Timeless.

"Not a bad life is it?"

"Hey, you talking to me or trying to convince yourself?"

"Bit of both I 'spose."

"Well suppose you hand me a cold one and don't be lagging on those chord changes."

I could go on. I could move the scene and the character and replace one race for another, one song, one sunset, one island. It wouldn't make much difference. We had some damn good times. We weren't royalty but there were times when we felt like it.

An athlete is affected by success, or the perception of success, in many ways. For those who use sports as a meal ticket out of a lower socioeconomic existence, money in the bank is the critical marker. For those in less publicized, lower-income sports, like triathlon, the measure of one's achievement must come in another form.

When I look back, yes, I see the hard times and the work, but I also remember the debauchery of the postrace parties, when a group of athletes with so much pent-up anxiety, so much energy and fitness and physicality, would take over a whole dance floor and just bust it out. There were many a night we closed the bars at 2:00 A.M. and went looking for someplace else. We were playing an unaccustomed role, putting off for a night our discipline and dedication. We'd dress up again as athletes in the morning. Talk about the benefits of being fit.

All these memories of such a heightened sense of existence—from the prerace tension, to the great performances, the disappointments, the crowd's roar of approval—you take them with you when you leave the sport. Like a beloved child or spouse, they are irreplaceable. You carry those memories around with you like a life raft. And like a ball and chain.

The raft can save you when everything else in your life sinks, which in some ways it must. How can you replace that feeling of having it all? You live by the memories, holding court at the local pub or surrounding yourself with people who will listen to your thirty-eighth rendition of the day you made that diving catch, or skated onto the Olympic team with that triple axel.

The best thing that can be said about memories, regardless of what you do with them, is that no one can ever take them away from you. People can criticize you, stereotype you, talk behind your back ("There goes someone who used to be..."), or worst of all, forget about you altogether, but they can never take your memory away. It is yours.

But memories are like fine china, a stunning totem of your position. You bring them out on special occasions to celebrate and to send a message to those gathered around you: You are special, share this with me. But if you use your fine china every day, maybe because you have come to depend on it, its significance changes. There is the distinct possibility that you are addicted to what it stands for.

That's the ball and chain part. Memories of youthful success, of game-wining touchdowns and gold medals and the roar of the crowd and a five-foot cardboard check for $10,000—those are part of a former life. You can and must savor them, but to dwell in them continuously is to live chained to the past.

"You awake Raymond?"

"Naw, just soaking it all in bro. Just soaking it all in."

I was lying on a beach of small cobblestones somewhere on the North Island of New Zealand with one of my best friends in the sport, Ray Browning. It was the day after one of the dozens of all-day Ironman events we would participate in during our careers. Our bodies were wrecked from the effort, out hearts and minds satisfied beyond anything considered normal.

"Hey, you see that little island out there? I think I'm going to swim around it."

Ray did not look at me as if I were nuts, as if I were being too competitive, or even as if he doubted I could make the two-mile round-trip through some rough surf. He never asked why. He knew.

F. Scott Fitzgerald said, "There are no second acts in American lives." Ray knew that we would never again be sitting on this out-of-the-way beach, less than eighteen hours after a one-two finish in a major event, in the best shape of our lives, the little rock island playing the part of metaphorical opportunity.

Ray knew that athletes get big chances, some of their own making, others by fate. He knew that you have to grab them, make them part of that memory. As those chances slip, so does the athlete.

"I didn't bring goggles."

"I brought an extra pair."

"You lead on the way out, I'll bring it home."

"Assuming you can stay with me."

"Hey, you aren't going to go writing about this are you? Because no one will believe it."

"No dude. This one's just for us."

▼ ▼ ▼

If you are a musician, you understand rhythm. If you live a simple life that revolves around the sun and the tides and winds, you understand rhythm. In our sound-bite, instant gratification, hard-wired world, we find it harder to live by any sense of natural timing and rhythm. Corporate punch clocks and deadlines just aren't the same as seasons and migrating geese.

The athlete must know rhythm. It is the undercurrent that they come to learn, depend on, and finally covet. The rhythm is an insistence of the march of time, providing the athlete comfort and security. It is not the same as day-to-day drudgery, where the task rarely changes or challenges. The athlete's rhythm stems from knowing the internal and external seasons of his or her career, of his or her body.

I could always count on a long, hard group ride on Wednesdays. I could count on running the trails fast with a few friends on Tuesdays. I could count on being exhausted the day after an Ironman event, but I knew I would still do something outrageous as a form of rebellious release.

Scott Molina, arguably the best all-around triathlete in the history of the sport, often had trouble with the Ironman distance. But he could suffer well, and for a number of years we had an unspoken agreement that we would play tennis the morning after every Ironman.

Now, you have to realize that most competitors have great trouble walking down stairs the morning after an eight- to twelve-hour race. Most times we were no different. But there we were, limping from net to backcourt, not because we really enjoyed it but because we could. It was just something we did. Rhythm. Predictability. Tradition.

Other competitors would walk by on their way to some fancy brunch and see us out there, flailing at a backhand and then massaging a calf cramp, and we knew they thought we were nuts. But we knew they would remember this strange ritual, shake their heads, and somehow understand the need to keep doing something once you start it.

Our season was long, March to October, or year-round if you wanted to race in the Southern Hemisphere during the winter. And during the eight-month season were distinct phases within each month, each week, each workout, and each race. Even though there were large similarities in training across each micro- and macro-cycle, there was enough creative opportunity to keep things new and fresh, so that the same damn 5,000-yard pool workout you had done fifty times before could still seem novel. It is like painting in oil on a twelve- by fourteen-inch canvas: The size and medium are the same, but the possibilities are limitless.

In *A Fan's Note*, Frederick Exley sums up the well-defined existence of the athlete: "In football, a man was asked to do a difficult and brutal job, and he either did it or got out. There was nothing rhetorical or vague about it." And even if Exley's football player had clouded his life by a dropped pass or failed field goal, there was always next week and another chance to raise his ego and reinforce his identity as an athlete.

This clearly defined state of flux is part of why the athletic life is so attractive. An athlete always seems to be in a state of movement, rising or falling, on his way up or down—but never sideways. The smarter ones know it could all go away in a heartbeat, with a torn ligament or a public indiscretion. You work very hard for the spot, but nothing is guaranteed. "Only one day in the big leagues," the Walter Mittys will say, "and I can die happy." But the only true guarantee is that you will die.

Most athletes have some sense of the great ambiguity of their situation. They take comfort in the predictability of another season. They also know that in the world of professional sports, chance itself is predictable; an injury, an illness, burnout, age, mortality—they all carry with them some degree of probability. In pro sport, ignorance can be blissful.

Neither a two-mile swim nor two sets of tennis would be considered a smart move in the recovery process on the heels of a very destructive athletic endeavor. There would be other races. Why jeopardize them? We were pros, earning a living off those sore and tired limbs. Pros, intelligent enough to know that doing stupid things might be the smartest thing at that perfect moment in time. As paradoxical as that sounds, it's true. It's not so much "living for the moment" as it is the realization and foresight that being a pro athlete offers some interesting opportunities, life chances that are not to be ignored simply for the sake of the next competitive event. Because one day you'll retire and you can't make sense of this new puzzle of normality that everyone else has been living in.

Even though I had been studying, writing, teaching, and coaching in varying degrees as I retired, it was three full years before I finally worked a regular fifty hour week, showing up at a job Monday through Friday from eight to five. It was only a summer gig teaching junior lifeguards, wonderfully rewarding in some ways, but as tiring as logging four hundred miles swimming, cycling, and running.

By the fifth week I was beat and would fall asleep by nine o'clock at night. I was the old man, chasing seventy five kids up and down the beach, out through the surf and back in. One day I made the mistake of opening my mouth to complain about a sore back from too much time bouncing around in the rescue boat. The incoming flak I took from the fit twenty year olds was sharp, powerful and deserved. How many times had I dished it out to those who just couldn't "pull" when I was at the top of my game? This wasn't really the kind of job you complained about. It was a *gift*, as was my previous job. From then on, I took a few aspirin, lifted a few more eights, appreciated the great kids I had to work with and kept my mouth shut.

Every transition out of sport is different. That too, needs to be said more than once.

In his 1989 autobiography, *Out of Bounds*, Jim Brown discusses why he left football:

"There is no single tidy explanation why I left football...Straight out of football, I earned more money than I did in it. And no one tried to bust my head. I wasn't retiring from football, I was retiring from football to go into acting. I knew that if I went from stardom to something obscure, the descent was too radical, knew a lot of guys freaked when the adulation screeched to a stop. I was too hardened for that...it was good to be the King."

I don't know if "hardened" is the right word. "Savvy" or "insightful" seem more appropriate. In any case, Brown, always outspoken and controversial, knew some things about retiring athletes that many intellectual types did not: It's good to be king, if only for a while.

When you're playing with the best, at the top, and you know it, you have a chance to create history. You can become famous or infamous. The ones who can decide the difference sit in the press boxes and write about you, about your performance, about your personal life. They can decide your fate. People write stories about you, not always complimentary. It's nothing personal, the journalists say, it's their job.

"In America," continues Jim Brown, "the media is God...It doesn't matter who you are. The media will KICK YOUR ASS...You can't wage war on the media and you shouldn't. If you're famous, the media is there to exploit you. If you're smart, you can use it. You have to know the rules, play by them."

The first time I won the Ironman World Championships in 1982, I was thrilled but I had no concept of media rules. While the actual *feeling* of running that last two hundred yards down the now-famous Alii Drive wasn't quite as natural and complete as it had been the year before when I finished third, it was my most successful moment in sport since I began playing Little League baseball in 1964.

The lead announcer/commentary guy from ABC's *Wide World of Sports* was a gentleman named Jim Lampley. As soon as I crossed the finish line he put his arm around me and tried to pull me into the dramatic climax of the event. It was a classic media strategy: Get the winners right away while they are still tired, out of breath, and filled with unnamable emotions of fulfillment and bliss.

The problem for Lampley was that, given my huge lead in the race, I knew I was going to win. And as a former runner, I naturally did what runners do after crossing the line—I went to warm down with a short jog.

Looking back on the scene now, I feel a mix of guilt, glee, and wonder. I can still see Jim Lampley's face, his mouth twisted a bit at the sides, not very happy with me as I excused myself and said I'd be back in a minute. He must have wondered to himself, How weird are these triathletes, that after nine and a half hours of racing in the heat and humidity they feel the need to "warm down"?

This was my big moment; millions of television viewers would judge me on the words I chose in the next thirty seconds. And I went away to walk it off.

When I came back, Lampley, to his credit, was patiently gracious and asked me what I had done differently in training to move up from third the year before to the victor's spot.

"I learned how to ride a bike," I said in all honesty, not realizing how glib and self-effacing it sounded.

Good reporters love good stories. This was not one of them. Still, the media love noteworthy performances and the surrounding human drama. When an athlete does something heroic, the action itself communicates feeling and the story practically writes itself. People love to read about heroic feats; it gives them an image onto which to project themselves, an image of a person they are not.

If an athlete makes a mistake, especially off the field, the journalists also love it. People love to read about deviant behavior in their heroes—drug busts or gambling, for instance. It brings the athletes closer to the fans, makes them more real, more palpable. The fans say, "Wow, Big Jim Smith can hit sixty-eight home runs and still get caught cheating on his wife. He can be unreal and real at the same time. Just like life. Just like me."

It is difficult for the average person to appreciate just how much exposure the public athlete gets. If you are playing basketball with four friends and you miss an easy shot and follow it up with a string of four-letter epithets and a ball slammed into the ground, only those four guys hear your rant. When a player from a top college team or the NBA does the same thing, add five, six, or even seven zeros to the four or five witnesses and look for a short clip of the miss on ESPN that night.

When you're playing at the top of sport, everybody is watching. Your life is lived in a fishbowl. And if the bowl is small enough and you swim around for too many years, after a while it's not you inside that bowl but a manufactured image of what you once were. When you retire and they release you back into the sea, you wonder who is being released—the original fish or the clone?

▼ ▼ ▼

Some of the better players in the high-profile sports like basketball, baseball, football, hockey, tennis, and golf make a lot of money. The truth is, the amounts are sick—LeBron James's $90 million Reebok contract, George Foreman's five-year, $137.5 million deal with Salton, Tiger Woods's five-year Nike deal worth $100 million. And for many of them, it's not even the money, it's just another way of keeping score. I mean, it has to be hard to *spend* that kind of dough! Then again, athletes seem to find a way.

While I was putting myself through college, I applied for and received a government grant aimed at low-income students. I was awarded $3,000, tax-free, to be used for books, tuition, and lodging. I had been working hard at two jobs making about $50 a week, and all of a sudden I was living like a king. I had a 1967 VW that ran fine, an apartment near the beach that I shared with a great roommate, two surfboards, a bike with air in the tires, and a guitar with six unbroken strings. Life was good.

At the peak of my career I probably earned close to $200,000 one year. I remember figuring that, if I was still in that apartment, driving that cool little bug, I could have lived for ten years without working on that one year's salary, adjusted for taxes and inflation. I was no happier making good money; if anything, my life had gotten too complicated—the more I had to spend, the more it seems I needed. And when I retired, and almost all my sponsorships dried up except the most loyal companies, my income decreased by 90%: One full zero was lopped off. I found a certain freedom in downsizing; I liked not having to think about whether or not we could afford new carpets. My wife and kids did not befriend the cutbacks as I did. They hadn't known really tough times, and it was a source of stress for us. But I think that it was valuable in many ways, and I'm glad that I invested what I could, when I could, so that I had the luxury of a few years to go to school and get my graduate degrees and learn how to feel and how to write and how to clean the carpets instead of ordering new ones.

Keep in mind that for every Tiger Woods who earns over $50 million per *year* in endorsements, there are hundreds of extremely talented athletes in lesser-known sports doing equally incredible feats and being compensated with a discount on equipment—if they are lucky. The winner of the 2002 Hawaiian Ironman World Championship was awarded $100,000, a small payout considering the time and effort it requires to win. When I first won that event in 1982, I was given a nice trophy carved out of indigenous koa wood. When I won it again in 1985, the organizers had upgraded; my trophy was a triangle of Plexiglas. I figure that in the twenty straight years I competed in that race, the amount of money I earned directly from the event just about paid for my trips to Hawaii, give or take a few mai tais. And I am glad for that. While I certainly could use the hundred grand right now, I wonder what it would have done to my ego back then. Athletes, like fans and most members of society, have come to equate financial remuneration with talent, charisma, achievement, and to some degree, heroism. That's one reason for the top-heavy distribution of prize money in races: First place often wins several times more than second place because the media pick up on it and splash around the huge number, which generates more interest, more sponsor dollars, and even larger purses. Caught in the middle are the young athletes who see these figures and dream of making more money for two or three hours of competition than their parents will all year. Caught in the middle are the athletes from obscure sports who hang on to the dream that one day their sport will be *discovered* and they too can "pull down some long dough." Caught in the middle are the ones who are pretty good but not quite good enough to make the money cut. But they keep playing, sometimes until they are thirty or thirty-five years old. And they still are just living on the fringe.

And caught in the biggest web are those who earn the big bucks, get used to earning them, and begin to equate their sense of self-worth with their exorbitant earnings. Then they leave the sport and it all goes away, or most of it anyway. And they have to deal with the unraveling of everything that was built upon that financial house of cards. Where is the "character building" in sport then? That's why many kids were pushed into sport by their parents in the first place—to learn about life through sport. For the pros, it often works the other way around: The athlete fully understands his or her role in sport only after being thrown back into regular life.

The anecdotes are many that detail the financial demise of a once rich and famous athlete. Boxing legend Sonny Liston (who many believe was murdered as payback for some shady Las Vegas deal gone bad) was working as an enforcer for loan sharks at the time of his death. Some athletes are smarter or luckier, and end up with a few bucks to kick around in their later years. When the boxer George Foreman finally retired for good in late 1997, he was paid $5 million for a bout against Shannon Briggs, who was only paid $400,000. Before the fight Briggs said he "felt like he was going to the death chair." Foreman said, "You can only make so many millions...I'm not going to cry. I've got four sons out there and I'm not going to cry like a baby.

Back in 1987 I was as broke as a goat. The only reason I came back to boxing was because I wanted to make money to fund my George Foreman Youth and Community Center. I did that. I was able to give out scholarships. What more could I ask for?"

Foreman seemed in control of his life, his finances, and his future. He used boxing, instead of the reverse. He knew that sport can develop all sides of an individual. The key is keeping your relationship with sport in context: It's only for a while, it won't last forever. And all the money that you can make, well, it may buy you an ego boost for a while, but in the end it will probably run out, taken from you by opportunistic businessmen, groupies, and your own blindness to the fact that money has nothing to do with your wholeness as a person.

What You Lose, What You Miss

*"A lot of things had intruded on my innocence and the boy
I was. I struggle every day to get back to that place."*
—Don Henley, musician

This is what you will miss when you retire from a life in professional sport: You will miss having excuses for everything you don't want to do. It's quite easy, really. They're automatic. Your sport comes first. Drive to your mother-in-law's? Sorry, I have a long training ride lined up. Take the kids to the dentist? Are you kidding? That's when I run, when I have batting practice, when I get a massage, when I lift weights, when I take a nap.

Yes, you will miss those easy excuses. Not only did you get used to making them, but now the people you unloaded them on will want you to make up for lost time. They will want their fair share. They will want a revenge of sorts.

You will miss the smells, the smell of fresh-cut grass hanging in the air on a late afternoon in early April. And you will hear a man in a restaurant say to his friend, "Do you smell it?"

"What?"

"Baseball, that smell is baseball."

And as long as you live, you will know that smell and exactly what he means.

You will miss the smell of oils and lotions and balms and creams—one or two for every purpose in sport. Balms to warm you up, creams to cool you down, lotions to keep the sun off, oils to help other things soak in. You will miss these smells because of what they mean, what they represent. The olfactory sense is considered the most powerful of all the senses. Smelling conjures up more images, more personal reflections, than hearing or seeing or touching or tasting. Smells are memories.

Every time I smell Irish Spring soap I am reminded of a guy I laughed with, who could make fun of me and build up my ego in the same sentence. I don't miss that smell but I miss that friend, Bill Smith, the champion's father, the man holding court at every race headquarters hotel bar in every city on the tour, a fixture at every race that mattered. I miss Bill Smith.

When his son Spencer first went out on tour with us, he wasn't even old enough to rent a car. But he was so good he bought a brand new Mercedes within eighteen months. His father Bill was loud, proud, protective, and gregarious. The father went everywhere in tow, making sure his boy was as primed and ready as possible. Most twenty-year-old kids would have been embarrassed by a dad like that. Not Spencer, though. He knew people were talking behind his back. But he loved his dad unconditionally; he let him shave the hair off his back so he could swim faster, watched him work well into the night as he tweaked and tuned his only son's bike to perfection, watched him argue with officials over an unfair call. And all these things Bill Smith would do for any other competitor if asked.

I walked by a group of young pros one day near the end of my tenure and overheard one kid I'd never really liked bad-mouthing Bill. He was the type who had things come easy for him, who expected things to be done for him when he had accomplished very little in his short career. He was a "trustafarian," a trust-funder who wore his hair long and pretended to know the meaning of *Irie*. Something in me snapped.

I hadn't been in a fistfight since sixth grade; I was a pacifist who had applied for conscientious objector status. But when I heard this kid say, "Spencer's old man is a pain in the ass. You guys see the way he dotes on his kid?" all those years of wishing my dad had seen me race, of watching my own kids clap when I ran by, wishing they could see me cross the finish line first just one more time, wishing I wasn't six minutes behind the leader—it all came out and I went at this punk. Slowly at first, I gained momentum as I moved in close, ignoring the "What's up grandpa Tinman?" I grabbed his shirt collar, just like on TV (it seemed uncomfortably natural, although I'd never done it before), and I put my face two inches from his, ignoring the obvious fact that he outweighed me by twenty-five pounds and could probably put me down with one swing. But I had a hidden rage at the world, at unfairness, at loss, and it was deepened by the image of a father and son traveling the world like drinking buddies, with respectful love, unmediated, uninterrupted love.

"You bad-mouth Spencer's dad again, I'll fuckin' hurt you, hurt you bad."

He thought I was joking and said, "What's up grandpa? You going to try and break into the top ten in the women's race tomorrow?"

I cocked my right arm like a bowman pulling back the string. He still didn't get it, and all the guys at the table laughed except one who saw it in my eyes. He stood up, moved between us, and told me it was cool. The kid didn't mean it. He was young, naive, stupid.

As I walked away I realized he was right; the kid probably had a dad who didn't care. I was just as naive and stupid for thinking that violence would make everything right. But I wasn't as young.

Neither was Bill Smith. Two months later he was diagnosed with brain cancer. Six months later he was dead. I miss him, and in my weaker moments, when I smell Irish Spring soap, I wish I had broken the trustafarian's nose.

You will miss the smell of gunpowder, though the smell of gunpowder is different. Gunpowder reminds me of outdoor awards ceremonies and fireworks, back when a few hundred bucks spent on some oversized bottle rockets made everybody feel better about how they'd done at the event, and resolve to do it again next year.

You will miss the freebies. Not the cars or trips to Hawaii you earned if you were good enough or lucky enough to win. But the little things, like bartenders telling you that last drink was on the house, you played well tonight, or the owner of the restaurant telling you that your money is no good here, that his kid has three posters of you hanging up in his room.

You will miss the fame, the kudos, the applause. That is a sound that will come back to you in your dreams and in your everyday life. That sound of people putting their hands together meant that you were liked, loved, appreciated. Eventually, it came to mean that your life was worth something.

There is a poignant tale in baseball folklore that involves the great Mickey Mantle during his later years. As the story goes, Mantle was spotted by a young reporter in the lobby of a hotel, alone, staring out the window and listening to the rain on the panes of glass. Approached by the reporter, the usually distant Mantle turned to him and said, "Listen. It sounds just like applause, doesn't it?"

Retired athletes everywhere, in their most honest moments, will speak of a sense of absence when the cheering died. They will have different names for their new condition—the pit, the netherworld, purgatory, or as my friend Kenny Souza called it, "the silence of un-comfortability."

Former pro athletes will often try to replace this "appreciation," "recognition," and "love." The avenues they choose are as varied as the individuals themselves. But even success in other aspects of life, whether in business, family, or politics, can't quite replace the imme-diate closeness and gratification of applause.

When I stopped racing a lot, I began playing my guitar more. I wrote a few songs, practiced them, and tried to convince myself that my voice wasn't that bad.

One day I signed up to play my songs at a local coffee shop. I in-vited no one; I simply took my case and told my family that I was going out for a bit. It was one of those "open mike" nights, usually a slow Tuesday or Wednesday when nobody was around and people would just show up, sign up for a fifteen-minute slot, and take their shot at a Warholian slice of fame. You could sing, recite poetry, read from your diary, or extol your political ideologies. No holds barred. But most everybody sang and played an instrument. That was the standard of-fering, especially if you were halfway decent, which I wasn't.

There were only seven or eight people sitting around, talking among themselves, sipping coffee or reading the newspaper. It wasn't exactly an opening act for a major band. Still, I was nervous. I wanted to be accepted, appreciated, even admired, if only for having the courage to get up and play. I wanted all those things I used to feel when I stood on the podium at the awards ceremony after a big race.

I played one song, poorly, stopping before the final verse because the coffee grinder in the back, I imagined, was providing more of what the patrons wanted. I sat on the stool and looked down at my reflection in the beautiful polished spruce of my acoustic guitar. When I moved the instrument slightly my face disappeared; it seemed to represent everything that was missing in my life. I put my guitar in its case and got up to leave. No one had even glanced up to see me sitting in the corner, singing a song I had written about—what else—love gone bad.

As I walked out of the coffee shop, a man sitting with his date lifted his eyes to meet mine. He wore a tight-fitting shirt and had toothpaste teeth, straight and white. His hair was perfect. Secretly, I wanted him to stand up and ask me if I was Scott Tinley and then tell me that he had followed my career, and that it was great that I could come and play a song without having a huge entourage around me. But all he did was look back at his girl, smile those perfect teeth, and forget me as I walked out.

I felt as if someone had torched the ground beneath me. I was on fire and all they could offer was a small cup of ice. I figured that when pain exceeds pleasure, get the hell out.

There are retired athletes who have followed an artistic path with some degree of success. And they do it for reasons that have nothing to do with the terrifying sound of no one clapping.

Tim Flannery played eleven seasons as a well-liked, scrappy utility man in the San Diego Padres baseball organization, never with more than a one-year contract. This was before minimum salary requirements, before the big dough. He didn't retire rich. But he was ready to leave, not knowing what he'd miss; if anything, the pain had exceeded the pleasure.

Always a fan of music and an amateur singer-songwriter, Flannery turned to music with the work ethic that made him popular with the fans. In recent years he has improved greatly, occasionally selling out small, intimate venues. Tim was a good ballplayer. He is a good musician who has learned to surround himself with better ones. His two careers are linked in ways he may never be able to explain, other than to say that it feels good to play, to be appreciated for a talent.

The famous child psychologist and former president of the British Psychoanalytical Society, D. W. Winnicott wrote in his landmark book *Playing and Reality*, "It is in playing and only in playing that the individual child or adult is able to be creative and to use the whole personality, and it is only in being creative that the individual discovers the self."

As much as the world of pro sports appears highly physical and workmanlike, there is a huge element of creativity in sport. The athlete creates poetry, emotion, courage, failure, and success from nothing but a period of time between the words "play ball" and the last out. When you leave sport, that desire and need for creation has to be channeled somewhere, somehow.

"Did you go to the music to find what you lost, what you missed in baseball?" I asked Flannery.

"Not really. Music is something I *need* to do. It's healing, it's creative, and the performing is a validation of all the work and preparation needed to put on a good show."

I sat there listening, trying to maintain the old separations: left brain/right brain, physical/cerebral, hard/soft. In the end I decided they weren't all that different, maybe on some level no different at all. Flannery played baseball for himself. He plays music for himself. In the game of life, a player without a game is dead. Flannery's music helps keep him alive. If he could never play guitar and sing again, he would miss it like hell. Maybe more than baseball.

If you have sport in your life it also serves as a release valve of sorts, easing the pain of loss. I started running around the time my dad died a tragic death of cancer in 1972. And I haven't stopped.

Not too long ago, a reporter who was interviewing me told me that he had added up all the miles I had swum, run, and ridden in my career.

"Why'd you do that?" I asked.

"I'm not sure," he said. "I'm a journalist, it's our job to do those sorts of things."

"Well, how far did I go?"

"Conservatively, Scott, I figure your training has taken you to the moon and partway back."

"Well, how far back? Was I close to reaching earth or just out of the moon's pull?"

"If my math is correct, you made it just to the point where reentry into the earth's atmosphere burned up so many early spacecraft."

I wondered what I had missed while traveling through my own space of trail, road, and water. Had the journey been a wonderful experience? Or was it an escape, a hideaway from the heavy burdens of life? A creative venture, or just a job? In the end I decided it was all of that and more.

For Flannery, who lost his own father in 1999 (and who may have covered a similar distance chasing down fly balls and rounding the bases), music was a way of healing.

"My music," he says, recalling the days he sat and watched his father suffer from Alzheimer's, "was the only way of connecting with him then."

Flannery was a preacher's son. And apples don't fall far from the tree.

The autograph is the talisman of fame. I can remember sitting at the big sporting goods trade shows facing a stack of two hundred posters on a table and a line of people waiting for them, not long but a line nonetheless. Every tenth person, the empathetic ones looking to relate to the athlete as a fellow human, not up but across, would ask, "Is your hand getting tired by now?"

I would always spend an extra moment with these people, ask them where they were from, whether they followed triathlon. And later in my career, when the lines were much smaller, if there were lines at all, and the stack of posters moved slowly now, like my arms and legs, I would think that I should be worried that my hand wasn't getting tired from signing autographs.

Be careful what you wish for, fuckin' superstar.

The irascible tennis great John McEnroe used to label adult autograph hounds "pathetic individuals." Even in his most obnoxious moments, though, the temperamental star always had a kind word, a signature, a disarming smile for the kids. Only the hardest, most cynical athletes are unaffected when a kid comes up to them on the street, maybe after a game, and asks for an autograph from his favorite player. Athletes may not enjoy this at the time if they are trying to find some peace and quiet, but someday they will. If they have a heart beating inside them, they will miss that.

The superstars, the really great athletes, will be interrupted at dinner and in the grocery store and while talking to friends. Out of earshot of the press, the stars will grumble how tired they are of "those intrusive fans." But later, as the fan's memory dims and the athlete starts to look back on his accomplishments, the scale balances; then the athlete will welcome a kind stranger reminding him of the time he hit a three-pointer in the playoffs, or ran the last four hundred meters in fifty-five seconds.

You won't miss the prerace jitters, the uncomfortable dread that sits in the back of your gut like bad news waiting to be told. "Butterflies" is a misnomer. You feel fear: fear of loss, fear of failure, fear of errors and dropped balls and cramps, of getting old and slow and losing your spot on the team. No, you will not miss the anxiety of fear. But you will remember what it feels like, its shape and color and texture, just as you will remember the victories. Those you miss so badly it hurts.

Winning is *not* a statistic—a simple fact of life—as maybe a thousand people have told you. Winning is a drug, a powerful force that reveals the best and worst of our species. The need to win pulls you in like earth's gravity, slowly at first but increasingly stronger the closer you get to its core. No player is immune.

The great cyclist and three-time Tour de France winner Greg LeMond wanted to keep winning at something so bad that he switched to a new sport after illness and injury forced him to retire before he was ready. It's not uncommon. LeMond tried his hand at car racing, spending hundreds of thousands of dollars of his own money trying to recreate what he had as America's premier cyclist of the 1980s and early '90s.

Eric Heiden took his five Olympic gold medals from speed skating, put them in a drawer, and did very well at bike racing. National motocross champion Jeff Ward worked his way up the ladder in car racing and just missed winning the Indianapolis 500, eventually finishing third.

All of them were letting go but holding on, moving on but standing still, dying and being reborn.

With great pain and years of effort, the addiction can be controlled, put away in some dark recess of the mind. But as with any addiction, you can't bring it out and play with it. You might reshape it, hide it under the guise of some business venture, as many athletes do, but once you are shackled by that feeling of hearing your name chanted by the crowd, of seeing your name on the scoreboard, of beating all the others—the chains may slacken but they never break.

To say an ex-pro misses the victories is like saying an alcoholic misses his or her drink. They tell you they are reformed, that they don't need it any more, that they are glad to be out from under the weight of addiction. But they miss it. Every athlete misses winning.

You will miss the *regularity* of things, the nice, neat package your life had been wrapped up in. You knew what you had to do every day. Either someone told you or you convinced yourself that a certain *order* was needed in your life if you were to succeed. You knew what to eat, when to work out, what time the bus would pick you up, how many shoes to have your sponsor send, how many races were left in the season, how many people were ranked above and below you.

At the same time, you will miss the spontaneity, or at least the ability to be spontaneous. When you are a pro athlete, much of the off-season is your own. You are strong, fit, confident. You need to express a few things bottled up since you began the last season.

Tom Warren, the reclusive and enigmatic winner of the 1979 Hawaiian Ironman, was always spontaneous, even during his serious training periods. He would ride his bike from his home in San Diego to Los Angeles and back in a day, just to drop off a piece of mail to a friend.

"Couldn't find a stamp," he'd say and then ride south, leaving the friend standing at the doorway shaking his head. If he knew Tom, he'd close the door and chuckle in admiration, knowing that some of it was just for effect. Still, he would be impressed at the iconic figure as he thought of his day's pedal.

Warren might run the fifty miles to Mexico and back just to be able to tell a friend when asked about his day, "Just ran to Tijuana and back; nothing difficult." Or he might do a thousand sit-ups in a sauna on a bet. Warren is the kind of athlete who defies description, who balances out the PR-trained, sound-bit, pre-fab, hair-gelled, jocks that we tire of. Athletes like Warren are increasingly rare. Today's pro sports have little tolerance or use for them other than as subjects of little vignettes on late-night cable sports shows.

Warren's most quietly momentous stand may have come while he and a girlfriend were making a three-mile passage between two small islands in the lower Caribbean on a ferry.

"It was really hot and crowded," he recalled. "Man, they had jammed way too many people on this boat, so I was sitting up on the rail trying get some air, giving my girlfriend more space. Then the captain comes on the loudspeaker, a real arrogant dude, and tells me if I don't get down off the rail he'll make me swim the whole way across. I looked at the distance and the tides, figured it was only 'bout two miles, and stayed up on that rail.

"Then the captain comes back and starts screaming obscenities, threatens to have me thrown off the boat. The people around, just as frustrated with the crowds as I was, looked at me in a challenging way, like, well, get down and make him shut up or start swimming.

"So I took off my T-shirt and shorts—I had a Speedo on underneath—pulled my goggles out of my backpack and jumped over. I'm sure my girlfriend never doubted it. The poor passengers though. It took them three times as long 'cause the boat had to follow my swim."

I, for one, miss the Tom Warrens of the sporting world.

Regularity, off the wall shit—my whole career was a series of black and white, polar opposites. When you're a pro athlete, your emotions are vertical: up when you win, down when you lose; building up for another season, winding down after the last. There is no vagueness. There is no need, no time, and no requirement to consider things of global importance.

For a time, I trained with a younger group, faster, stronger "kids" who I latched onto in hopes of staving off Father Time just a few more years. Kenny Souza, a little speedster, a hard working, wonderfully big-hearted guy with street smarts but not much more than a high school education, was one of the rabbits I chased around on the bike all day. When we did slow down enough to have a conversation, it invariably centered on triathlons, competitors, equipment, or the odd vicissitudes of racing for a living.

One day Kenny asked me, "Hey, what was that Vietnam thing about anyway? I've been meaning to ask you. I used to think it was a new restaurant. You didn't go fight in a war before you were a triathlete, did you?"

No, Kenny. I missed it by a few slim years. It wasn't my war anyways. I knew I couldn't hide out under the insulation of pro sports much longer. I needed to expose myself to the world. And that nakedness can kill an athlete's career.

"Wow, man. But racing, it's sort of like war anyway, you know, when you want to kick someone's ass and stuff," Kenny said, trying to figure it out.

Well, negative motivators are not healthy, I thought. But I stayed within my own thoughts, recaptured by the blanket of ignorance, ignoring the outside world, telling Kenny to focus on the next hill. The Nam was a long time ago. People much smarter than us will never understand.

You will miss the clarity of training, when you could embrace and measure the day by reading from your training log. You will miss the fight, not the constant struggle to make it, but the real and illusory battles played out—fought—between the starting gun and the finish banner. I suppose I could say that man is born to compete, drop some Darwinian notion that we really have no choice. But that would be wrong. Our world is well populated with nonaggressive Ghandi-esque types; an entire generation, it seemed, filled the streets in the late '60s. And yes, it is possible to be a peace-loving athlete. Just unusual.

But I was able to find a struggle, a war against something inside me powerful enough to motivate and propel myself through a dozen years of forty-hour training weeks. All athletes define their inner battles in a way that drives them to fight on the outside when the competition begins. And when those inner battles have been fought, and the dying embers of that fire fail to yield the same heat, the athlete's career is over. You can redefine it, play for enjoyment, try to make the quintessential "comeback," but it can never be the same war. And you will miss the war.

"Football players and athletes generally get into this kind of being or beingness," former NFL quarterback John Brodie once told the author Michael Murphy in trying to describe a state of mind many athletes strive to play in. "But they often lose it after a game or a season is over. They often don't have a workable philosophy or understanding to support the kind of thing they get into while they are playing...But during the game they come way up. A missing ingredient for many people, I guess, is that they don't have a supporting philosophy or discipline for a better life."

If sport provides you with that heightened sense of existence, and it goes away, you will go searching for it—even if you can grasp the connection between sport and a more basic need to do battle. You will miss sport because you felt so alive when you played. And when you feel "dead," the desire to feel alive will grow so strong that it will make you do crazy things, things that normal people will consider extreme, dangerous, or anti-social.

Still, even with all the feelings of loss and the pain of coming down—of dying, as Goethe said, so that we can live again—most of us would do it again in a heartbeat, and miss it every day for the rest of our lives.

Part Three

▼ ▼ ▼ ▼

NOT ANOTHER DAY IN PARADISE

When It's Time

"You never really have the opportunity to grow up. It's like you're living in a candy store and nobody tells you that you'll ruin your appetite."

—Alan Page, NFL Hall of Famer and Associate Justice of the Minnesota Supreme Court

ords—worrisome, threatening, dark, and reflective— I couldn't get away from them. As I threw myself into studying athlete retirement, many times it occurred to me that aging is like the water that freezes within a rock and splits it apart: It doesn't happen on purpose, it just happens.

When my career track finally made that bend in the road, that slight turn toward the place I was headed, the words of warning kept coming at me.

I'd see quotes in magazines and newspapers I wasn't even used to reading. I'd hear portions of conversations that had relevance to change, to transition, even to death. And I'd stop everything I was doing and listen. I'd walk out of bookstores with books on sociology and philosophy of sport. I began reading difficult academic texts on anthropology, mythology, and social psychology. Subconsciously I knew my ability to go fast on a bike, on my feet, between two black lane lines in a pool, was waning. The only place I was going fast was into the vacuum where my identity had been.

For some reason I thought the constellation of possibilities beyond the finish line would be made clear in the words of those who had gone before me. I could not have been more wrong.

I looked for stories, guidance, and hard information on athlete retirement: how to un-become what you have been for so long.

Nothing.

I had always had other interests besides sport, even when I was at the top of my game. I had helped launch a successful line of performance athletic clothing with a few friends. I was doing some public speaking, camps, clinics, videos. I had written two "how-to" books on triathlon and a couple more that dealt with some of the more esoteric and intangible aspects of sport; only one of these suggesting that I had promise as a writer, but they sold well nonetheless. Despite our differences in schedule, background, and ideology, I was still married to the only woman I had ever considered as a lifetime mate. We had two kids together and we wanted to give our best shot at raising them well.

I just wasn't worried about what the opportunities might be when I quit. There were no signs that I was going to lose my sense of who and what I was. I knew there would be some catching up to do, as I had been living inside my own dream—and, as I realize now, other people's dreams too. But even though the extracurricular activities I had dabbled in were a nice diversion to give me a sense of balance in my life, they were not the same as living through each and every stage that an individual must pass through as he or she grows up and, with luck, grows old.

What I wanted to know, what every professional athlete wants to know, is: When is the *right* time to hang 'em up, to quit the damn game, and deal with all the shit you never had to?

Some fans argue a star should quit at the top of his game; for them, seeing a former star failing at what used to come effortlessly is like watching a man dig his own grave. Others, like the writer Rich Cohen, feel differently.

"In my opinion," he wrote in *Harper's*, "a superstar has an obligation to play until he can play no more, until the tank runs dry and the wheels burn...The great player must suffer through his wane with a kind of grace, for only in the end can you see his true character."

Cohen may not have played professional sport, but he appears to understand that the end, not the beginning, is the hardest. Just the opposite of an individual retiring from corporate life.

After forty years with the firm, a sixty-five-year-old man or woman is ready to live out his or her life on the back nine with a tall scotch and soda waiting on the veranda. A thirty-year-old middle linebacker retiring with bad knees has forty or fifty years left to live, not ten or fifteen. How is he going to fill them up with meaningful activities, with something that makes him feel needed and wanted? How is he ever going to replace what he has lost: the sound of thousands cheering, the sense of being unstoppable, impenetrable, the best in the world. How is an athlete supposed to rediscover *that* selling cars or doing commentary for TV or playing golf with the old playing buds, swapping tales from hole to hole? As Jerry Sherk of the Cleveland Browns once told me, "The sooner an athlete realizes the best part of his life is over, the sooner he will begin to heal from that tremendous blow."

In 1996 the NFL Players Association approved a Ball State University study that would focus on retired players' health. One of the facts uncovered was that of the 1,425 retired players contacted, two thirds had left football with a permanent injury.

"For years every player in the league thought he would die at fifty-five," said Mickey Yaris-Davis, the director of benefits for the NFL Players Association, who likened that fear to the urban legend about alligators in the sewer. The problem was not longevity, he added, it was quality of life. "These guys retire at thirty-five with ninety-year-old knees. Imagine what they'll be like at sixty-five."

Actually for a quarterback, the haunting number is thirty-eight. Dan Marino, John Elway, Joe Montana, and Steve Young all retired at thirty-eight. Johnny Unitas had Achilles tendon surgery at thirty-eight. Sammy Baugh broke his hand in the preseason after turning thirty-eight and retired the next year. And the indefatigable George Blanda, who stayed in the league as a kicker for the Raiders, gave up most of his former quarterbacking duties with Houston when he turned thirty-eight. Few quarterbacks were very productive after that age, the exception being Warren Moon who played until he was forty-four.

"No one wants to see his hero," wrote Cohen in *Harper's*, "the idealized image of himself, become tired and old. With the first hint of decline, the first sad steps down the mountain, the Superstar is urged to 'Go out on top,' a useless phrase that only diminishes the connection between sports and life; in life, no one goes out on top." No one that is, who doesn't die an early, violent death.

By the mid 1990s, I had missed my chance to go out on top. My first sad steps gave way to a precipitous fall from where I once was. But I didn't care. In fact, it became my own private battle cry. I was almost forty years old and still fighting to finish in the top ten of a few big events. At times I felt a need to give something back to the sport, but I didn't *know* most of the young pros. We hadn't sweated blood on a thousand training runs and rides together; some seemed arrogant, like they wanted all these benefits but they had no patience. So, when I beat them in a race, I would purposely hustle over to the beer tent, grab a few cold ones and come back to the finish line, barely able to stand, and act like it was just another long training day for me. The hard part for me was realizing that not everyone admired you for what you had accomplished. Maybe I had put too much faith in humanity, but when it hit me that there was a degree of resentment and envy over the fact that I was still out there, my anger rose at first, then waned, and finally turned into depression. Not only would I not go out on top, I might end up going out on the bottom, a pitiful shell that head-shaking critics would point at, forgetting to say how good he once was. Some smart-ass in the background would be mumbling that you're only as good as your last race. And he would be right.

On occasion I would have a respectable race and think, okay, not bad. I can still bring it when all my stars are aligned. But that was my former self talking shit because he was afraid he was going to get dropped when the future stepped in.

At least I appeared to have the good fortune of leaving the sport completely on my own accord, when I wanted—if I ever did completely. Doug Williams, the first African-American quarterback to win a Super Bowl (he was also named Super Bowl MVP), knows about when it's time.

"The drum beats for everyone," he once said. "No matter who you are, there's going to come a time your career is over and you'd better be ready for it."

It is more of a problem for the team player to "abandon" his or her sport, even if they feel they are abandoned by it. If a lifelong football player retires but still loves *playing* the game, what are his options? What would Johnny Unitas, arguably the greatest quarterback to play the game, have said if one Sunday morning he woke up and felt like playing a game of touch football? Could he get on the phone, let the word out that the Great Johnny U wanted some? And would his aging knees even allow him to take a snap and drop back in real-time slow motion, each and every hit he had ever taken from a 240-pound linebacker rising up from his past? Could he get off a short loft to a neighbor's kid on the sidelines? Could he fight his arthritic demons with a memory? Would throwing a few spirals after lunch with his grandson be enough? Having something you love taken away, even if you walk away from the crime with your head high and a case full of trophies, is still a theft. You are still leaving, and you can never stand in the same river of gold twice. Some things you bury, must be buried alive.

After I won my second Ironman in 1985, I decided to watch the telecast of the show. I had always had a hard time watching the Ironman on television. The early TV producers had taken something that for me was so raw and elemental and made it into something orchestrated and mediated, just to hold the viewers in their chairs and sell them cars and soft drinks.

But I was the winner of that delayed broadcast and I was curious to see how I was portrayed. Besides, I was out of town, at a trade show in Dallas and wanted an excuse to go to a health club to work out and "watch the show." So I parked myself on one of those early Exercycles lined up around the tube and convinced the other cycling viewers to let me switch off the golf match just for a minute to watch "a race where all the chicks rode their bikes in their bikinis."

I pulled my sweatshirt hood up tight around my face and watched the standard formula unfold: scenes of palm trees and volcanoes, some human-interest stuff, a helicopter shot of the long ribbon of asphalt that makes up the course, an update on the leaders, more human-interest material, a break to the national ice dancing championship, and then a final return for an interview with the winner by some B-grade commentator.

But what struck me was the conversation vectoring around the room among the other viewers, weekend warriors who were close enough that I could smell last night's garlic shrimp oozing out of their pores, spewing a "What the hell is this Jimmy? I thought you had the golf on."

"Oh, it's that thing in Hawaii where they swim through lava and run like fifty miles or some crazy thing."

"Is that the leader there? Boy, the fella sure seems small for…what'd you call it? An Ironman?"

"Yeah, he's some cocky California kid, seems like he's got it in the bag. The kid's got a ten-minute lead and he's smiling and joking with the camera guys on motorcycles."

"How could he be so fresh after a whole day of all that exercising? That doesn't seem normal."

"Larry, when you were in the steam room the kid was playing football while he ran. Like I said, one of those West Coast hippie-jocks with long hair."

"I thought you said it was swimming, biking, and running."

"It is. Somebody from the media threw a football at him and he was tossing back spirals to the sound guy while running seven-minute miles."

"Now that's something. I don't know whether he's nuts or some abomination, but the kid ought to retire soon as he crosses that finish line. How many of us would trade our soul to the devil to get on national television throwing spirals?"

The show ended and I had an anonymous shower and went back to my hotel wondering if my life indeed had reached an apex. Yes, I won easily because most of the top guys weren't there; they were still nursing sore legs from a big race in Nice, France two weeks prior where I had finished second. And yes, I had thrown a football back and forth with a guy from the TV truck while I was running. But no, I finally decided, I wouldn't hang it up there. And they weren't solid spirals; they had wobbled just a bit.

Each sport has its own exit paradigm, its own ways of letting you go, kicking you out, keeping you in, or drawing you back. I thought my style of a slow, gentle exit, "gracefully surrendering the things of youth," would be the least traumatic. After I stopped winning major events, I still had good sponsors. When I failed to make the top three, then the top five, I was still a well-known triathlete, invited and paid to come to events around the world. But finally, after a gradual decline in my competitive accomplishments over six or seven years, after I entered my first race in twenty-five years checking the category box on the race application labeled "40–45" instead of "professional," I knew what it felt like to be buried alive. Time and stress and gravity and life itself were doing the shoveling. I was watching my body decline from the pinnacle of physical fitness to a body that might, well…it just might do OK in the forty to forty-five age group.

It's funny. No, it's sad. I wonder how I could be so hard on myself. I'd take that age group-winning fitness now. And this is from a guy who was pissed off when he finished second at the Ironman four times. I'd take that now too.

While it was hard to move slowly off that peak, ironically, it was good for my health. Even though it would take me a full three years to reach a point of basic health, with a strong immune system and hormonal balance, I could feel my body returning to its normal state from before I began serious endurance training. Of course I didn't appreciate this at the time; my guilt over slower track times distracted me from the benefits of the new homeostasis.

I wondered about the timing of other athletes' retirements. I knew that single-sport athletes like me, who had already paid the price of the solitary training, who had already invested in the Bank of the Long Lonely Mile, found it easier to keep playing or training.

A runner needs only his shoes and the air to breathe; a cyclist needs only a bike and a stretch of road or trail. Indeed, it is refreshing to see a former pro play just for the love of the sport. How encouraging to hear tales of a retired Michael Jordan organizing a pickup game of hoops with his buds. Athletes who play for the "right" reasons, based on some higher-order motive than fame or fortune, never leave completely. A part of them may still want to play, but at that moment of epiphany the bigger part, or at least the physical part, says, "That's it. I'm over it. Move on. My heart's not in it."

And sometimes that bigger part is a busted part.

Greg Welch, a World Triathlon and Hawaiian Ironman Champion, was hit by nearly all of those at once. He loved nothing more than to swim, ride, and run with his friends and wife. He had been doing it for the right reasons. But he didn't get to plan his exit. In fact, he barely kept his life, not so much betrayed by the sport as ambushed by his total enjoyment of it.

It began in late 1998, the last year he had any real motivation to train. Something deep inside told him that he had accomplished everything he had ever hoped for. But the sport of triathlon would be making its Olympic debut in the Sydney Games of 2000, and being the most famous and successful triathlete in Australia, Welch really didn't have a choice—he *had* to be on the starting line in the shadow of the Sydney Opera House.

From a competitive standpoint, his 1999 racing season was very encouraging. He won a number of events around the world and was an easy favorite to make the Australian Olympic triathlon team. But Welch, a carefree, easygoing kid from a small town south of Sydney known for its good surf and tall eucalyptus groves, wasn't doing well with the pressure.

"I felt very stressed about making the Olympic team," Welch recalls. "I was looking for any excuse not to make the team; setting myself up for failure knowing full well that my talent and potential could put me there."

Those who knew Greg well could sense this. He was slower to laugh, his hair began to thin on top, his jokes seemed forced. But what could anyone say? Welchy, as he is known, was preparing for the Olympic Games, which would be held in a city just a short bike ride from where he grew up. A medal in these games and he wouldn't have to worry about a thing for the rest of his life—Australia reveres its sport heroes like no other country I've seen. Free beer for life for me matey Welchy.

The worry, though, the thought of not standing atop that podium under the Sydney Harbor Bridge, may have been his undoing.

No one can ever say if the problems with Greg's heart that began during the 1999 Hawaiian Ironman were stress induced. It would be a futile investigation for Greg to undertake. Let someone else be the subject of that research. Welchy has to go on living first.

It's called ventricular tachycardia: the rapid, unstimulated acceleration of the heartbeat into the dangerous range. And now, after two years, two dozen operations, and more pricks and prods than any man should be party to, Greg Welch walks around with a little watch-sized defibrillator sewn into his upper chest. If his heart should jump from a resting rate of 55 to 255 beats per minute while he is playing with his kids or sound asleep, the lump in his chest will send out a shock that is supposed to "reset" the rhythm. So far it has only happened once, when Welch was pushing his one-year-old daughter across a busy street. The shock sent him flying while he desperately hung onto the handle of the stroller. That was the fastest Welchy has moved in the three years since he retired.

"I tried to be something that I wasn't," he says in a wistful voice. "I put pressures on myself that I couldn't handle. I was ready to leave the sport, but I felt a sense of duty, a sense of commitment to see it through for all those who had supported me in the early years." Welch had given everything, including his lighthearted personality, the kind of person he had been. A year before the Olympics he was teetering on the edge, dancing out in that zone where every great athlete must live for periods of time. But just when Welch was figuring out how to step back gracefully, he fell.

The search for that elusive better life, even after you find what you thought you were looking for, can blind you to what it was that you really wanted. Sometimes you have to step back and watch your exit as if you were watching yourself in a play or a dream, removed enough from reality that your interpretations and your choices can be more objective.

In this the athlete is not unlike an artist: Writers and painters often return to their work after having set it down and left it alone for a period. And upon viewing it with "fresh eyes," they begin not to re-form their work, but to hone it, tweak it, mold it closer to the expression that they want to make.

Some players need to remove themselves from *any* contact with their sport as they create a new identity. The psychologists call this "reaction formation." It's what teenagers do when they act as if they hate their parents. It's what the writer Mark Twain was talking about when he said, "When I was sixteen I thought my father was the dumbest guy around. But by the time I turned twenty-one, I was surprised at how much the old man had learned."

I think I needed a distant vantage point to see clearly what triathlon had meant to me from my first race in 1976 until I left the pro ranks in 2001. I may have had the wisdom of the years inside me, but it sometimes takes a while for that wisdom to assume a form and shape that can be passed on.

Retirement is like a marriage or a divorce: You never really know what it's going to be like until you do it. Oh, you can think on it all day, pay it so much mind it will drive you crazy. But in the end, it's a combination of what you make it and what it's going to be anyway.

NFL star Ronnie Lott thought about it, so did the baseball great Nolan Ryan.

"I used to talk all the time to guys who had retired," Lott told writer Bill Lyon, "asking them how they felt, how it felt to be out of the game. I have the philosophy that you should never assume that life is going to be what people think it is."

Indeed.

And Nolan Ryan, an ageless icon who kept throwing no-hitters at an age when most guys were ten years past their prime—an intelligent man who could out-think the smartest hitters—even Ryan apparently saw the wisdom of stepping away for a period.

"I always thought there was going to be life after baseball," he said in his induction speech at the Hall of Fame. "I didn't realize the grip baseball had on me. It took me two full years to get over the fact that I was no longer a baseball player."

But Ryan is a baseball player. He cannot bury his past any more than he could have predicted his feelings upon retirement.

The great tennis player and political activist Arthur Ashe, considered as insightful, intelligent, deep-thinking, and considerate as any athlete of our day, a man who once said in reference to his fight against AIDS, "Believing that pain has a purpose, I do not question either its place in the universe or my fate in becoming so familiar with pain"— even he had his moment of confusion in transition out of sport.

"One life had ended," he says in his autobiography, *Days of Grace*, "and another had not yet quite begun...I had to negotiate the middle passage between the old and new...At this crucial point in my life, I did not want to make any major mistakes."

Nobody does. But Ashe applied some of the skills he took from tennis; he gave his life direction and form.

"I had known this moment would come, but now it was here in earnest...Quite consciously, I gave myself a period of about three months simply to think about the past and about the future."

It appears that Ashe embraced his retirement willingly; he stepped out of one skin, one uniform, stood naked before the world as he pondered, and then began moving, one step at a time. There was no denial, no dream of comeback. Perhaps he had a sense of loss, but Ashe's emergence into a newer, more intellectual, spiritual world, a world where he would give more than he would take, aided his transition.

How ironic that the sporting world would experience its own deep loss when AIDS took the life of Arthur Ashe when he was fifty years old. I know it's a damn cliché but it still is true: The good, they die young.

When the Time Has Passed: A Player's Pathos

"A denial of one's wounds is like the denial of one's life—it ends in premature death. A lived life is one that not only looks at wounds but embraces them and follows them like road signs."

—Jim MacLaren, writer, speaker,
and former top amputee athlete

T he wondrous Nolan Ryan might have been surprised by the grip baseball had on him. But over the years, he has loosened that grip, as we all must, one finger at a time. And he is far from alone in the experience.

The tennis great Bjorn Borg once said, "It wasn't until I stopped playing tennis that I realized that in real life problems exist." And they do. When the athlete retires, that same grip remains, holding as hard and fast as the athlete grips back. You can't stay. But you can't leave. And the worst part is when the choice is made for you. Greg Welch had the choice made for him. So did three-time Tour de France winner, Greg LeMond.

LeMond had already won the biggest bike race in the world, arguably the toughest sporting event of the modern era. He had won the World Championship in 1983 and then, still in his mid twenties, he finished the Tour in third place and then in second before finally winning in 1986. Most experts picked him as the favorite to win for at least another three years.

Professional cycling has history in Europe. Several million people line the small country roads to get but a momentary glimpse of the Tour riders as the large pack pedals by at jersey-blurring speeds. In America the most people knew of cycling was what they learned watching the movie *Breaking Away*. LeMond was changing all that. He was the thin, fair-haired boy from Reno, California, who moved to Europe on his own, was signed by a European team, and began to attract attention over there—and finally over here.

Sadly, he was not noticed by his brother-in-law as he crouched low and tight against a small clump of bushes while they hunted turkey and pheasant. The brother-in-law mistook the moving bush for a pack of pheasants and sent LeMond to the hospital, bleeding from a dozen holes gouged out by a shotgun blast, proving that no one is immune from life's tough blows.

While LeMond regained his form in one of the greatest comebacks in the history of sport, winning the Tour de France another two times, his fortunes changed again. There's LeMond, on the heels of that great comeback, winning another two Tour titles, but starting to struggle.

"I was constantly fatigued," he said. "I started to doubt myself, doubt my training, my nutrition, my technique. It caused a lot of confusion. I had been to every type of specialist there was, and no one could find anything. There were so many doubters, all these people saying that I was looking for an excuse to retire. Heck, I had two more Tour wins in my legs. What did they know?"

Of course they knew nothing, nothing but shallow human emotion. Greg was still a young man, still an athlete with the skill and determination to win another Tour. He knew he could. What he didn't know was that the lead left in his body from the hunting accident was causing a rare muscle disease that had no effect when he rode his bike up to the corner for a six-pack but would not allow him to scale the Alps or the Pyrenees with the best riders in the world.

"I was actually quite relieved to find out that my problem was a medical one, not in my head," he said.

"Did it make it any easier?" I asked him.

"Well, it wasn't the type of retirement I envisioned."

Of the twenty Hawaiian Ironman World Championships I competed in, I finished all but one. Like LeMond, I had something wrong with me physically, something the docs hadn't found yet. But I was a lab rat: Nobody was doing what I had been doing for all those years without a break. It shouldn't have taken months of testing in the best labs in the country to figure out I was burning the candle at both ends and in the middle—with a blowtorch. I could have saved myself years of pain and grief by listening to my mother. She started in when I was in my mid-to-late thirties. "Scotty, don't you think you've done enough? Aren't you ready for something else? Your body must be…tired."

But I didn't listen. I had worked too hard to get there. I was going to milk this ride, dammit. I was going to ride it until they scraped me from the side of the road with a spatula and said, He's done, take him away. If the birth of wisdom is the emerging concept of the obvious, it was about to hatch.

In 1996, two days before my fortieth birthday, I was competing in my seventeenth straight Hawaiian Ironman Championship. I had trained hard. I was in shape and I wanted to make a point, mostly to myself, that age was just a number. I could do anything better at forty than I could at twenty: solve math problems, surf, make love, swim, write poetry, change a flat tire, or build a fort for my kids. It took me longer to recover from hard training and racing, but I ignored that minor detail and pushed through; there'd be time enough to rest when I was in my eighties. To prove it, three weeks before the race I had picked out my high school mile record time of 4:42 and run three of them in a row with three minutes rest. Screw time. I was ready, burning my tires in preparation. This dog would hunt.

But time has a way of playing tricks on us all. I started the race slow that year, hoping to pick up momentum, but I slipped from the top ten to the top twenty; at mile twelve of the marathon I was barely inside the top forty, and the slightest ray of wisdom peeked into my head. I sat down on the side of the road. There was gas in the tank, the tires were new, but my carburetor jets were bad. No fuel was getting to the muscles. I knew I was digging my hole deeper and deeper. So I quit, just turned around, stuck out my thumb, and waited for a ride back into town.

As I sat there, the leader Mark Allen ran by on his way back into town. Behind him was an armada of media vehicles and people on bikes; it was a parade of human drama and Mark was the Pied Piper. "Nice job Mark," I said and tried to read his eyes, but they were focused well into something that only he could know. Maybe it was the finish line, maybe it was heaven or maybe they were turned back on themselves and all he saw was his own space and time, hearing only the sound of his breathing and his heart beating like a perfect drum. And for just a moment I felt jealous. I didn't like the feeling though. I wanted to be in the lead of the Ironman one more time, with a five-minute lead and three miles to go, my legs pistoning up and down, my wet shoes squishing in sync with the sound of camera helicopters above, signaling the end of the pain and the beginning of the celebration. But Mark and his army of well-wishers passed, leaving me to wonder if I should try and walk the last sixteen miles of the marathon. How long would that take? Would it hurt me? What were the costs? The benefits? Did it matter? Did I really care if I kept my streak alive or was this a nice excuse to abandon what might become a burden of a different type in years to come?

As I sat there in contemplation, a solitary figure on a moped passed, slowed, and then turned around and came back. It was a race official and he recognized me from years, maybe even decades, past. He didn't say anything, but he saw the hurt in my face, the disappointment dripping out from behind my Oakleys.

"Here," he said just above a whisper, "hop on and I'll give you a ride into town."

As we passed Mark Allen, now less than a mile from the finish line and beginning to dismantle his fortress of concentration, I threw the jealousy away. He had more than earned it. I was happy for him. Self-pity hath no room in my heart. Begone bitch.

That night I wandered over to the bar that sits above the finish line. Normally it's a restaurant with a nice ocean view where the tourists watch Kona Bay sunsets and sip umbrella drinks. On race day, though, it turns into an evolving hot spot: omelettes at the race start for VIPs, rum drinks at the end as the middle-of-the-pack finishers run the last one hundred floodlit yards down Alii Drive, the Holy

Grail of triathlon. The bouncer recognized me and let me in, "Eh, brah, you always welcome here in Kona. No matta you drop out." I wanted to go back to my hotel, put my shoes on, and finish the race—just because this man had said the right thing at the right time.

Instead, I walked upstairs and immediately ran into a familiar face. "Tinley, get over here you skinny surf punk! What are you drinking? Hey bartender, two margaritas for the two-time champ!" It was Greg LeMond, just having finished his TV commentary duties. He handed me a drink, took one for himself, and said, "You don't need to say anything."

"But..."

"Hey Tinman, who do you think you're talking to?"

Then there's Tim Flannery, the guy who retired happy, having given everything he could to the game. A guy who was "motivated by fear of failure," he would say. "Whatever it takes to play, I'll do." A guy with a self-admitted obsessive-compulsive drive who retired at thirty-two years old after playing the last two seasons in a state of constant pain. He had some difficulties in transition but after a few years he found himself back coaching in the minor leagues, and then as the third base coach for the San Diego Padres. Flannery says that regrets are a curse. He's right.

Flannery knew better than most that the role of the professional athlete has changed in recent years. He knew that athletes are entertainers, that their value to the team owners is in entertaining the paying fans, winning games, and doing something heroic if the opportunity presents itself. Tim was a realist with a family to feed. As much as he disliked it, he could play the political game and still keep his integrity intact. He'd always have his music.

On the morning of his forty-fifth birthday, he was fired from his job with the Padres organization with one year left on his contract. Flannery was quoted in the local paper as saying, "I love this organization. I love the manager, and I love the front office." The general manager from that front office was quoted as saying, "He probably needed a break."

The Padres finished last that year. The message on Flannery's answering machine later that same day said he would not be available for a few weeks. He would be off "healing."

Athletes sometimes have to wait before they are willing or able to say what they really feel about their retirement. Sometimes it's at a Hall of Fame induction ceremony, as they grasp the last prize the press could ever hold over them. Sometimes it's just sitting around with a bunch of other retired jocks, swapping tales about how good they were, the lies not really lies because they actually did all those things.

It might happen on an all-sport talk show, well scripted in advance, but still a memory sneaks past the security door and the "on air" signs. And there it is: Some profound revelation about the unenviable task of having to recreate yourself at age twenty-five or thirty-five or forty-five. Even the most cautious and private are not immune. It must be part of the healing to say out loud, "Man, it hurt. I was a damn mess when I quit," or to make an observation so powerful and clear that it will silence the most seasoned reporter or fan. And you didn't even mean to.

Even the great Los Angeles Dodgers pitcher Sandy Koufax, arguably the best left-hander in the history of baseball and a man intensely protective of his privacy, could slip, but only once. Chapter 1 of his autobiography ended with this enlightened group of words: "An athletic existence is a self-liquidating life."

If we say that the athlete's body is a ticking clock, then retirement is a bomb. Sometimes you decide to set it off, sometimes fate sets it off early, but the fuse is always burning. You can watch it burn down and do everything possible to delay the inevitable explosion—eat right, work harder, learn yoga, wear baggy shorts—whatever it takes to feel young so you can play young. Even as you watch the flame move into the body, still denying it will affect you. But sooner or later it goes off.

I remember Women's PGA Hall of Famer Nancy Lopez, the holder of forty-eight tournament wins, trying to qualify for the U.S. Women's Open in 2002 at age forty-four. But a six-over-par seventy-eight in a qualifying tournament sent her back to the practice tee. One of the greatest golfers in history broke down in tears on the eighteenth green and told the reporters, "I'll just have to find something else to do."

Most of the public would feel an instant connection to Lopez. They too have failed at something they used to take for granted. A few might be less compassionate and think, "What, you're sad that you don't get to play golf in a tournament? Get real." Lopez's place in history is secure. What is not secure is the future. And the athlete, trained to handle physical challenges that would send most of us running for cover, is rarely trained for change.

But who is? Everybody deals with change, with transition. What about the guy who works for the same company for twenty-seven years and is "let go" three years before his retirement kicks in? What about the "empty nest" we spoke of, the mother who raises five kids on a shoestring, devoting her entire life, her entire being, to making sure that they walk out of the house with as many tools as possible to flourish; and when the last one kisses her on the cheek, says, "I love you Mom," and climbs on the bus headed for college—what about that mother? How do you compare these people to a professional athlete who "has to" retire because of a sore foot or because he can only run the forty-yard dash in 4.9 seconds? How do you compare Bjorn Borg, Tim Flannery, Nancy Lopez, or Greg LeMond with the Vietnam vet? One week he's caught in a firefight outside of Da Nang, the next he's shipped back to the "world," his tour of duty complete, and he finds himself sitting in front of the TV on his mother's couch in Illinois with a bottle of cheap bourbon and a bag of dope. They all feel detached from the reality that was their world. They all feel depressed, lonely—dead.

In some ways there is no real difference. Everybody has to deal with the trauma of change. In other ways, though, the unexpectedness, the compression, the hidden emotional pain, and the misunderstanding of the athlete retiring *do* represent something different. And so athletic retirement cannot be compared with or studied according to any established theory of loss without confusion.

Consider the tale of NBA Hall of Famer Bill Walton, an athlete who persevered through hundreds of injuries and dozens of operations. A highly intelligent and creative person, a man with a family, he seemed ready to do whatever he wanted after he left basketball.

"How did you formulate your plan?" I asked him one day.

"I had no plan."

"Nothing?"

"Nothing."

I find his response hard to believe, but I listen carefully as he revisits some of the crossroads he faced, the fortunes he uncovered not in money or fame but in family, friends, self-discovery, and contributing in newfound ways to a game he says he was "born to do, born to love."

You would expect a player like Walton—a member of Coach John Wooden's UCLA dynasty in the 1970s, a three-time winner of the NCAA Player of the Year award, the number one draft pick in 1974, a member of the Portland Trailblazers championship team in 1977, the MVP of the NBA in 1978, a smart man who graduated with honors from UCLA with a degree in history—well, you would think that he would know exactly where he was going after a career in the pros.

Where Bill Walton went was on tour with the Grateful Dead.

Always a free thinker, even considered "a bit radical for the NBA" by writers back in the late '70s, Walton seems almost as proud of his membership in the Grateful Dead Hall of Fame as he is of his place in the NBA Hall of Fame.

"Starting in high school, I started following rock and roll and the Dead in particular. But after meeting Mickey Hart and Jerry Garcia, I had the opportunity to travel with the band, sit backstage, and drum along. I went to over six hundred shows before Jerry died and the band dismantled. And all those guys from the band are still my best friends. That's what I did when I left the NBA."

When Walton left the league in 1985, after playing his final few years with the Boston Celtics, his body was not in good shape. He had undergone thirty-two operations to keep him playing in the NBA: two on his left hand, five on the left knee, and the rest on his problematic ankle, which in the end was fused in a 90° angle, effectively preventing him from ever running a real step for the rest of his life. Now it is commonly known that the medical advice Walton received was not in his best long-term interest. He was not born with the body type to play twenty years in the NBA—few are. But after a series of stress fractures that kept him from playing, he would eventually consent to treatment that kept him playing...temporarily.

"I don't hold anyone responsible," he reminisces, "I lived to play basketball. That's all in the past...Forgiveness sets you free."

Walton, who now enjoys a very successful career as a basketball sportscaster—he has won an Emmy Award for best live television sports broadcast—still has no idea what he would have done had he not followed a lead into broadcasting. He also doesn't know what he will do when his days behind the microphone come to an end.

"That day will come," Walton says, "and I will sit down and re-evaluate where I am and what my options and unfulfilled dreams are. When I was a player, I never made big plans for the future because I knew I would be a totally different person when that time came. The same thing will go for my next career. I expect my life will change radically again, and I certainly hope to be doing this for a long time because I truly love it."

Sounds to me exactly like a Grateful Dead concert: You follow a lead, a hunch, another band member's chord change and add your own story to it, because you're not really playing the same song as when you started five minutes or five hours ago. But over time, you've created a journey with a past, an unknown future, and a wild and wonderful present—a long, strange trip.

Finally there's Jerry Sherk, linebacker for the Cleveland Browns, graduate student of psychology, mentor of troubled youth, observer of the human condition, especially his own.

At times, we disconnect and see ourselves like a different person. It's not an out-of-body experience; rather, we have become depersonalized from the individual we used to know. The passage below was written by Sherk in the last days of his career almost twenty years ago.

I know that I am done. It is December, and I'm at the very end of my last NFL football season. After twelve years at defensive tackle, the knees have disintegrated and they can't take it any longer.

He uses the word "they" to refer to his knees, as if they are no longer a part of him. Sitting at the kitchen table with his journal, he pauses for a moment and raises his head as if to listen before beginning to write once again.

This big house is quiet and empty. I couldn't sleep so I am sitting downstairs at four in the morning, feeding my dogs, two Irish setters. There is a full moon and several inches of snow on the ground. My dogs don't question why I'm up at this hour, their only concern is to get at the full plate of scrambled eggs that I've just made for them. For some reason, I amuse myself that I have gone to the trouble to cook people food for my dogs. Perhaps it's the irony of sharing this time in my life with dogs instead of a woman.

He lifts his head again to watch the dogs finish licking the plate. As they sniff the floor for anything they may have missed, he thinks to himself, "If I smoked cigarettes, now would be a good time." He begins again.

Here I sit alone in this large home in the Ohio countryside, and through the window the moonlight reflects off the snow and illuminates the aspens and maples in the backyard. The beauty of it all is breathtaking. My thoughts go from this scene back to my life. The dream achieved, and it means almost nothing. What do I have—did I have? Where do I go next? What do I do? I still have some pride, a sense of accomplishment. But sitting here this morning and looking out the window, all I have is the reminder that I've come so far and achieved my dreams, only to know now that I stand on the edge of being no-thing.

He goes back and whispers the paragraph he has just written, and when he comes to the end he underlines *no-thing* and then says it out loud: "no-thing." Both dogs are now sleeping by his side, and the large male setter looks up to see if he's done something wrong before plopping his head back to the floor.

Without football, without my ability to express myself through football I am nobody. I will disappear. Football has been my life and I have so little else. All that is left are these two dogs, this empty house, and this moment in moonlight.

Pathos Plus

"When you stop playing the game, it's like dying."
—Tim Green, NFL player

This is what else happens when you retire from a life of high-level sport: You get lonely.

A great majority of the symptoms experienced and described by retired players can be traced back to loneliness. An athlete says he feels lost, disconnected, spacey; he tells you that "something is missing, but everything is fine." The words point to a loss. If you can get an ex-pro athlete to sit down and open his or her heart to you, to reveal what it is that they miss the most, do you know what often comes up first? The other players, the locker room banter, the camaraderie—that's what they miss the most. Big, strong men and women, some of the best physical examples of the human species. I know it was that way for me.

And why wouldn't they be lonely? Many pro athletes are adults trapped in childlike minds, insulated and protected by the team, the league, their families, and most of all their peers. Sport is fairly simple. The rules are well spelled out and you know what you have to do to improve, excel, and win.

Coaches, managers, doctors, and agents make sure that the player doesn't get too distracted, too far away from the task of winning games or events. It's a very black-and-white world, a perfect place for a young man or woman to stay young. Perfect for playing with your friends.

You love the sport because it loves you back. And you miss that love.

NBA Hall of Famer and basketball executive Jerry West once said, "This has been an incredible love for me. To even think about walking away from it, that's very painful." This is one of the primary reasons why so many players gravitate back to the game as coaches and managers. They want to stay connected to the game, to the players, to their passion, because it's what they know.

When NFL quarterback John Elway retired, he told *The Sporting News* that he felt like he had just gotten rid of a 2,000-pound load. Julie Krone, the most successful female jockey of all time, said she was going to spend a little time just sitting on the grass and looking at the sky.

"They teach you how to play the game," NHL icon Gordie Howe would say, "but they don't teach you how to leave it."

And then all three of these players would recast their thoughts later, realize what they were really saying was that the retirement might have seemed right at the time but brought with it confusion and lonliness.

What you may miss most of all is the person you once were, the person with that well-trained body that could do all those amazing things. High-level sport is nothing if not physical. Your body is your weapon of choice, your marketing vehicle, the carrier of your hopes and dreams. Your body is central and must be well cared for, pampered, prepped, and propped back up when knocked down. You are completely in touch with your body; your world could not be any more self-sensuous. But sooner or later the body changes. For good. You will miss it, and you will miss what it stood for.

When mine started to decline, I fought back. And I fought hard, which in endurance sports usually makes things worse. I fought my slower times like quicksand, shaking and squirming my way into an even faster rate of descent. The sad thing was that I knew better. I had been self-coached my entire career; I knew my body needed a long rest, not more intense training. But I was working against personality type. Acceptance was far off in the future, past denial, anger, bargaining, and depression.

I remember waking up one day when I was in my early forties and feeling like I had gone twelve rounds with a heavyweight. I had scheduled a long bike ride with a couple of young hotshots and I didn't want to get dropped. Out came all the stops: a hot-cold shower combo, double espresso with a shot of Kahlua, aspirin, the latest energy drink, a Power Bar, some yoga poses, and race wheels. I *never* trained with race wheels; that was cheating. But I needed to cheat somebody so I figured it might as well be myself.

Right then I needed to go back to bed—for a year. But my deluded view, empowered by the fear of losing what I once owned in my body, had occluded my intelligence. All I had left was a hammer. And the whole world looked liked a nail.

Athletes are used to controlling things. All it takes is an incredible amount of innate talent, years and years of intense training, and opportunity. Every time a race is won or a curveball is hit deep into right field, that sense of control is reinforced. That's what the fans see when the players make it look easy.

The more astute spectator knows well how much is behind every perfectly performed skating routine. They know that the nineteen-year-old girl who just scored 9.8 or 9.9 has been skating since long before she was eight or nine. To play at the top, you have to be able to control everything from nerves to muscle cramps to in-laws wanting free tickets to the Olympic finals.

When you retire, suddenly you don't get to control all aspects of your life. You certainly can try, as many do. It is hard to accept the truth that absolute control is simply an illusion. Sports propagate the illusion because they offer many opportunities for control and success.

John Elway, the winningest quarterback in NFL history, retired in 1999. It seemed a storybook ending. He had won the Super Bowl, invested in a number of interesting and promising business ventures, stayed married for eighteen years, and fathered four great kids. Elway had retired as a king, on his own terms, and it seemed he would remain in control.

Just over three years later, his world was upside down. His twin sister and his father had both passed away, many of his business ventures had gone sour, and his wife had moved out and taken the kids with her.

Elway, to his great credit, did not pull the covers up over his head and retreat into some dark space. In a *Sports Illustrated* article in August of 2002 he told journalist Rick Reilly, "When you're a quarterback, you're in control. The football's in your hand, and it's fourth-and-twelve, and if the wideout doesn't take the right route, I'm going to run around and make things happen. But now, things go wrong and I don't have the football anymore."

All too often, it takes this degree of pathos, of tragedy, for a successful and famous athlete to turn his or her attention inward for answers. Because the answers aren't as simple as they were in the pros.

There are a great many people who can bring pleasure to everyone but themselves. Often they are artists: painters, musicians, sculptors, writers. The best are gifted individuals who hone their craft to levels that amaze us, make us stand humble with admiration and ponder how such creative genius, such grace and power, can spring from the human species.

And many of them are tormented by their gifts, living lives that may appear idyllic from the outside but are filled with suffering and grief that can compromise or destroy the individual. They are somehow "different" from the everyman. And often there is a price for that difference.

There are great athletes in this group, athletes who sit atop the dais as we heap them with praise. They are the Van Goghs and Emily Dickinsons and Charlie Parkers of the sporting world. They are the best, but they are not happy.

Darryl Strawberry was one those, a brilliant ballplayer and by most accounts a kind and generous man, the type of person you might have a drink or a chat with and say to yourself, "What a great guy." But Strawberry could not make himself as happy as he made the fans and the people close to him, whom he gave cars and houses as gifts. He had more than one drink and spiraled down to that place where life is so raw and real that the illusions are muddied, and you face your demons knowing that you either learn about yourself—or die.

Strawberry's story is pure pathos. Like other athletes before and after him, he had it all and lost it all. And if you have but one ounce of compassion and understanding, you won't simply blame Darryl Strawberry for his addictions to drugs and his crime of using them. An argument could just as easily be made that our society's overemphasis on victory, the fans' need to get what they came for—the fans' dependency—are also responsible for Strawberry's woes.

Strawberry is guilty of a failure to possess that inner core of strength, that self-protective instinct that other great players have and use to avoid earthly temptations. Strawberry wanted to be accepted as much for who he was without a bat or mitt in his hand. But people wouldn't let him.

Indeed, Strawberry is guilty of being human, of having human faults.

"I never had a problem hitting. I had a problem living," he once told Michael Sokolove of the *New York Times Magazine*.

Like great artists, great athletes rarely have a true insight into their own lives while they are playing. There just isn't time. If they did, they might not like what they saw. And that would certainly play havoc with the task at hand—winning games and races and tournaments.

I asked an employee of International Management Group, the largest and most powerful athlete representation firm in the world, if they ever "counseled" the players under contract with them. "We're not in the psychology business," he told me. "Besides, a lot of these guys wouldn't like what we'd have to tell them."

No, the lucky ones think about it along the way, consider it while they're still playing the game. Most defer the process until their knees and backs are more suited for office chairs and couches.

"At some point," Elway told *Sports Illustrated*, "it hits you. This fairy tale life you've been leading is not real." But it is real because it happened. And now the athlete must face a new kind of reality.

What that new reality brings with it is old baggage, all the emotional shit you swept under the rug while you were too busy training, racing, traveling, doing photo shoots for the sponsors—too busy running toward something that could never end.

But it will come back—all that baggage, all that immaturity, all those unresolved questions of identity come back to you with the force of a three-hundred-pound linebacker.

The box is open now. And you can't put your emotional baggage back in. The best way through it is to play it straight up, honest, no more end runs, no more kidding yourself about playing another year or competing in just a few more races. The sooner you realize that your life may never be as exciting as it was, the sooner the healing begins.

When I discarded my professional athlete's protective shell, I hadn't really cried in twenty-five years. That first year, when my life was in transition and turmoil, I cried almost every day. Oh, I'd put up the strong front, rarely mention how I felt to anybody who I thought wouldn't understand, which was just about everybody I knew. But in the morning, after my wife left for work and I got the kids off to school, I'd come home to a quiet, empty house, a lonely house, and I would surround myself with all my books. I'd lie down on the couch in my office with Campbell and Schopenhauer and George Sheehan and D. W. Winnicott and Larry Brown and the Dalai Lama and Tim O'Brien and Rumi and Durkheim and the Bible and Twain. I'd just pile these books next to me like new friends and pick one up at a time, open to any page, and start reading. I was searching. I was coping.

For a while I didn't have a clue at what some of the deeper passages meant, but I figured it was better than drugs or alcohol, better than joining a cult, better than fooling myself into thinking I could be one of the best endurance athletes in the world again. Then something in one of my books would touch me, a passage, a poem, a painful scene that I had lived through but never fully processed. And I would cry, feeling a pain so deep and intense and unnamed that it would paralyze me. How could it be this bad? All I was doing was changing jobs.

But I could not have been more wrong. I was changing lives. I was shedding the skin that had grown around me over twenty-five years as an athlete, the clothes I had worn that kept me from having to deal with any problem that was remotely uncomfortable. You'd be surprised how many times I could dream up a long run or an ocean swim when my wife was pissed off or the kids were screaming. Or when I thought about my dad dying and leaving us all alone.

I purposely began reading books about father-son relationships, desperately seeking catharsis with each page. My life was unraveling, like it was supposed to.

I had rebelled when my dad died. I had watched that cancer eat away my hero one cell, one day at a time. Looking back now, I can say that my desire to become a professional athlete was not driven by ego or competition or money—it was driven by my need to rage against disease and normality. My dad had been a rebellious type as well, never allowing the myopic conservatism of the status quo to rein in his creative and free spirit. To him, everybody had a voice, an opinion, and should be given a chance. When I was growing up, whenever we got all the kids in the neighborhood together to play football or baseball at the school across the street, or hoops against the garage wall, inevitably my dad would come out to play and we'd all cheer, especially the younger ones. Because when Terry Tinley was playing, everybody played, not just the biggest or the best.

Now if I could earn a living as a pro triathlete, if I could get paid to compete in a sport that most people couldn't spell let alone describe, then I could in some way avenge my father's death and all those little guys who were cut from the team, who were picked last if at all. I would step out of the box, embody health and fitness as no other sport ever had, and live the dream of immortality. If I became one of the best athletes in a brand new, California-bred sport I helped create, I would essentially be telling the rest of the established, narrow-minded world to fuck off. Try and take this away from me bitch. Go ahead, try and outwork me, outlast me. You'll lose. I swear you'll lose.

Thoreau once said that the hardest battle any human will fight is to remain true to him or herself in a world that is trying its hardest to make us something else.

By living life on my terms as a professional athlete, I was doing that. But when that life went away, I had nothing left to rebel against. So I rebelled against myself. My body was alive but most everything else in me had gone searching for a lost fifteen-year-old who was looking for his dad to come home from the hospital, pick up the basketball from the bushes, and tell his boy, "I'm only spotting you three baskets because of the bandages. Take it out boy. Your old man beat the Big C."

I'll never know for sure if losing my dad at a particularly vulnerable period of my life contributed to what I felt when I left the sport. Or whether it was due to the other "losses" that coincided with my exit from sport: my grandmother dying; my first-born, love-of-my-life daughter reaching puberty and deciding she wanted little part of her dad as she developed her own identity; the troubles my wife Virginia and I had as she tried so hard to understand what I was going through but never really could; the loss of my physical fitness; our decision (subsequently abandoned) to move out of the home we had lived in for ten years; or a deeply repressed consideration of my own mortality that surfaced as I reached the exact age at which my dad died. Whatever the cause, the trapdoor feeling that sucked the life out of me was akin to what I imagine death must feel like for those who are privy to its impending arrival. I'll never know, and quite honestly I don't want to. I'm okay with accepting that I made it through to the other side.

When It's Time, Again

"You know how I realized when I was through with football? It was during the Cincinnati game. I didn't want to hurt anybody."

—Chip Oliver, professional football player

"I don't think I'll ever get over it. You get so used to being pampered and applauded all your life, and all of a sudden you're in your own living room watching someone else get all that."

—Baseball Hall of Famer Mickey Mantle

If you do an Internet search with the key words "athlete retirement," you will get several thousand websites. Among the first hundred or so, the ones "hit" most often, at least half will refer to Michael Jordan's multiple retirements and comebacks. This is not surprising, considering how popular Jordan has been in the past decade.

Athlete retirement is not a new topic. The fans had mixed feelings about seeing George Blanda playing for the Oakland Raiders at age forty-five, and Archie Moore fighting at fifty. Some laughed at Bjorn Borg's comeback and chuckled to themselves as they watched the ancient (for boxing) but still imposing figure of George Foreman fight his way back into financial independence throughout his forties.

But the fans were also profoundly moved when Nolan Ryan threw a no-hitter at age forty-one, and when the New York Rangers' forty-one-year-old captain Mark Messier came off the bench and rallied his team to a come-from-behind victory as only a seasoned vet like Messier can.

▼ ▼ ▼

When alpine skier Bill Johnson became the first American to win an Olympic gold medal in the downhill, he was immediately hailed as a wonder, a hard-living, fast-driving kamikaze who could back up his brash predictions. The fans overlooked his outlandish behavior because many of them, at some point in their youth, had been just as wild. But his shtick, complete with the SKI OR DIE tattoo on his bicep, wore thin. Bill Johnson had a hard time being the humble, gracious champion. His star faded until it simply burned out, and he spent nearly a decade working odd construction jobs, making fewer and fewer skiing-related appearances, and thinking about what it was like to be the fastest skier in the world, if only for a moment.

And then, in the midst of a building comeback at age thirty-nine, Bill Johnson fell. And it hurt him bad. It was the U.S. Alpine Championships in March 2001, where Johnson was starting thirty-third in a field of sixty-three. He was in a coma for three weeks and when he came to, he wasn't the same "life on the edge" man. Everything happened slower. Everything.

But the irony is that now, in his struggle to get his body and mental acuity back to normal, Bill Johnson has attained the hero status that eluded him after the gold medal was draped around his neck.

> *"The athlete approaches the end of his playing days the way old people approach death. But the athlete differs from the old person in that he must continue living."*
> —Bill Bradley, former New York
> Knicks forward and U.S. Senator

In the summer of 1999 I was still experiencing bouts of anxiety and feelings of disconnection and depression. I searched tirelessly for a physiological explanation for these feelings. Every few nights I would call up my physician friend Dr. P. Z. Pearce in Spokane and run another medical scenario by him: Maybe it's this, maybe it's that. I knew I had pushed my body to a point where only a few other athletes had gone before. I had been asking it to get up each morning and spend the majority of the day swimming, cycling, or running for close to twenty years without more than a week or two off each year. There had to be a reason for my feelings because, for all intents and purposes, I wasn't *retired*. I still had sponsorship contracts, I still competed in races. I just didn't see myself as a professional athlete anymore. It had become a job instead of a passion. *That* I didn't see. *That* was at the root of my neuroses.

P. Z. would listen to my well-intended but amateur self-diagnoses with the patience of a country doctor, which he is at heart. One night I called him all excited, thinking I'd found the source of my psychological symptoms.

"I got it P. Z., it's an overdose of the amino acid L-phenylalanine. I added up the amount I'm getting in all the supplements and vitamins I take, and it's one hundred times the recommended adult dosage. Look here, the symptoms are the same as what I've been feeling."

Dr. Pearce just listened and then said quietly, "Wow, S. T., that was a great try. I'm impressed. Yes, you should cut out some of those supplements but that disease only occurs in infants."

Dr. Pearce had me try a variety of SSRIs (selective serotonin re-uptake inhibitors), medications like Prozac, Zoloft, and Effexor, with the idea that it might help my depression, although he also had a theory that long-term overtraining had compromised my adrenal-pituitary axis, resulting in decreased levels of neurotransmitters. There was some medical as well as anecdotal evidence for this theory, but the meds were only marginally successful and after I had tried and properly tested every one on the market, I went off the anti-depressants.

One day, in an effort to slowly convince me that my illness had many components, including quite possibly a psychological one, P. Z. sent down a "Life Change Index" test, a list of approximately forty-five items covering major life changes, with the resulting stress of each assigned a certain number of points. The index starts with Death of a Spouse (100 points) and various life events follow. There was Death of Close Family Member at number four with 63 points. Change to Different Line of Work would get you 36 stress points, Retirement got 45, and Minor Violation of the Law carried 11.

"Take the test bro," he told me. "Let's see how you do."

So I listed all the recent changes in my life, added up the number to 375, and called him back. "How'd I do? Do I get an A?"

There was silence on the line while a scoring sheet came through the fax and I read the fine print.

"In the persons studied," it said, "79% became severely ill within a year if the changes occurring in life totaled over 300 points."

"All things considered," he said, "I think you're doing pretty well."

I was approaching the end of my athletic career the same way I might approach death: with absolute fear, denial, and plenty of rebellion. My fight, my rebellion, which had been outward (me against conformity), was now turned inward (me against my own death). Some of the elements of this dynamic were becoming clearer. I felt disconnected, foggy, and vacuous because I was projecting my own mortality, reliving my father's death and the guilt I harbored for not having done what I could to make his last year more comfortable. Sport is many things to the people who play it at the level I did. For me sport had served, among other things, as a giant Band-Aid. And now that the Band-Aid was coming off, all the pus of my last twenty years was oozing out.

"There's no easier way to make a living than as a pro athlete," said Bob Pettit, former St. Louis Hawks center. "Then all of a sudden, you wake up and realize you have to go to work for a living." The "job" that faced me between 1999 and 2003 was to heal myself. And in hindsight, I couldn't have done it without those I turned to, those who also had played the game.

One of those was Barbara Warren, the wife of an old friend, Tom Warren. Tom won the Hawaiian Ironman in 1979, long before anyone put much stock in endurance events. Barbara was an accomplished endurance athlete herself who had done one-hundred-mile running races and cross-country bicycle competitions. She had a thriving counseling practice and, in my mind, was well qualified for the conversations I would have with her about my feelings.

One day she sent me an e-mail that moved me quite deeply. In it she said, "The road you will travel is bumpy and narrow. Nevertheless, don't ever take the wide one. It only leads to the death of your spirit and soul...It is very hard to achieve the growth you want with your little human power. Allow something supernatural to transform you."

I thought about the "wide path." What could that be? A return to sport? An effort to put all the bad shit back in the box, to place a nice new Band-Aid over the hole that had opened in me? Or a life built upon the foundation I had in sport? I could always become a coach or do TV commentary, maybe be a race director or give clinics. Heck, lots of former athletes do that kind of stuff and are very happy to have a place in sport. I could have gone that route but my senses were telling me that the road in that direction was too wide. Do something narrow and hard, my inner voice was challenging me again. Go against the damn grain.

Okay, hotshot, so you're kind of screwed up right now, lost your bearings, your direction, your momentum. So, big deal. Move on. Last time I checked, you ain't dead. You milked that cow for a long time. Now you're holding the pail. Set it down hotshot. And step away from the udder.

"It's not that easy. If human existence can be reduced to meaning, what sport means to me is a question of purpose, not value."

Oh, been reading the heavy shit again, have you? No wonder Virginia gets on your case when you talk like that. Truth is, in sport you can't separate purpose and value. They're tied together. Your purpose is what you make of it. Your value is what they make of you. You have to get control of your life back.

"That's good but I was thinking just the opposite, that I need to let go a bit, ease up and let someone else drive for a while."

Feel the Force, eh Luke?

"Cute. I was thinking more that it's about the experience. That's what I miss—that *something* that elevated my life beyond the everyday routine. I want that sacred feeling that I could get in workouts or races. I crave it like a drug. But I doubt I'll find it in sport anymore. Maybe the arts. You think I could be a rock star?"

Oh puuuleeease. Hey you could always make a comeback. Everybody loves a comeback.

Indeed, many people do enjoy seeing an aging athlete come out of retirement. It gives the fans hope; the player seems like Roy Hobbes in Malamud's *The Natural* or Joe Hardy in *Damn Yankees,* even if these stories are fantastic. And while it may take some convincing, even the cynics must admit that when one of the great ones retires it is an occasion of great loss, both for the player and for the sport.

"I remember the last season I played," said baseball great Willie Mays. "I went home after a ball game one day, laid down on my bed, and the tears came to my eyes. How can you explain that?"

There will never be another Mays or another Jordan, Elway, Borg, or Gretzky. These guys are not athletes for the ages but for all time. Their exit marks a notch in the timeline of sport.

When an athlete makes a comeback—and mostly we're talking about the stars here, as journeyman players aren't given the opportunity to come back (perhaps a blessing in disguise)—it's usually a final swing for the fence. Maybe they left the game unfulfilled or maybe they miss the camaraderie, the glory, or living on the competitive edge where they can test themselves day in and day out. But always there is the element of redemption: Returning athletes must seek out and redeem themselves one more time, either in the eyes of the fans or, more likely, in their own. The fan is thus given a stay of execution. All hail, Michael's coming back to play another season.

James Thurber once wrote, "The majority of American males put themselves to sleep by striking out the batting order of the New York Yankees." If you have achieved an equivalent feat in another sport, you do not forget it easily. And like Tolkien's golden ring, the memory has a power over you. It draws you back, pulling with a force that will continue until you let it go, replace it with something else, or submit and try one more season, one more event. Just one.

My relationship with triathlon was like a love affair: If I didn't take it too seriously, it didn't have meaning. But I found out in the end that when I took it very seriously, it broke my heart. I remember the words of a brilliant schizophrenic reported to me by a friend: "Love is not a game," he told her, "and everybody plays it." Triathlon had become more than a game, and I had to figure out a way to stop playing.

What It Feels like to Lose It

"There are moments of glory that go beyond the human expectation, beyond the physical and emotional ability of the individual. Something unexplainable takes over and breathes life into the known life. One stands on the threshold of miracles that one cannot create voluntarily...Call it a state of grace, or an act of faith...or an act of God. It is there and the impossible becomes possible...The athlete goes beyond herself; she transcends the natural."

—Patsy Neal, *Sport and Identity*

Jack Nicholson wasn't crazy and neither was I. In *One Flew Over the Cuckoo's Nest,* Jack's character had been ripped off, ultimately. In one of the final scenes, they took his mind and his existence. They killed him without ending his life, and he was saner than his protectors.

The word sanity, from the Latin word *sanitas,* or health, is equated with mental equilibrium, a state of *normal* thoughts and feelings. To act sane is to practice sound judgment or reason. But it is still a relative state. *Normal* itself is only achieved when one adheres to the conventional standard, pattern, or type.

Perhaps you were thinking that I was going to ask, "Well, if we were all nuts, would that be *normal*? Would it be natural?" Maybe you knew that I was a Jimmy Buffett fan and was going to quote the line from his song "Margaritaville": "If we weren't all crazy, we would go insane."

Or maybe after reading the last three paragraphs, you're just not too sure about the writer himself.

There was a period when I wasn't quite sure myself. The last day I remember feeling normal was January 25, 1999. I was up at our little vacation cabin that sits high atop a hill on a lonely stretch of Central California coast, alone, naturally. I had just finished a decent run through the backcountry. The air had a nipply feel to it: not quite biting, more like a slow painful gnawing. The ocean was the color of cold blue steel, mysterious with a nervous surface to it that seemed to keep me on edge. I had to travel.

I decided to drive farther north to a little town that I had my eye on. I had often fantasized about living there, but my family had put up a solid resistance. Still, I had a few days off and I could dream. The frenetic pace of the city down south had my cells working overtime. I sometimes dreamt that parts of my body would look at each other and ask, *what the hell is he doing to us?* I wanted to be where many ex-professional athletes go when they retire—a place you can wrap your arms around and feel the slow, steady pulse of small town honesty, a non-threatening little ville with a good library and a decent coffee shop.

The change came on slowly but with the force of nature. There was no stopping it. It was destined to take away the automaticity of my life, to hold me down until I gave up and accepted all that I had done, all that I was, and all that I was created to be.

Of course I didn't know this at the time. All I knew was that when I came around a big sweeping left-hand turn on the 101, the King's Highway, *El Camino Real*, a rush of nausea swept over me like a rogue wave and I was left with my nerve endings dangling like live electric wires, severed yet powered still, swaying in the breeze, exposed.

My first thought was that I was hypoglycemic, that low blood sugar from too many short-chain carbohydrates was playing tricks on my brain. I had gone through a bout of reactive hypoglycemia in high school, just after the death of my father (at least that was my diagnosis then). My glucose tolerance test had come back borderline, and a more stable diet balanced by proteins and fats seemed to lessen the symptoms of tingling, confusion, and a very strange sense of "disconnection" from the world. At least that's how I remember it now. Then again, that bridge between then and now, both tumultuous periods of my life, broken in the middle, may someday render clarity if re-connected.

Frightened, I immediately pulled off the freeway and stopped at a convenience store for a jar of peanut butter and a tuna sandwich. In hindsight, I think this reaction was an early symptom of denial showing up in physical form, a veiled neurosis creeping under my skin without warning, explanation, or known cause. Still, it freaked me out. It was like having survived a car crash once in your life and then having someone tell you to hold on, here it comes again.

I headed to a friend's house in a nearby town. He wasn't home, but the idea of simply hiding under a blanket on his couch seemed safer than driving around terrified that I might run head-on into a sixteen-wheeler in some momentary fantastical breakdown of reality. I lay on his soft leather couch, my soul riding shotgun on my mind, both seeking purchase in a world that seemed to make sense on the outside. But the inside and the outside were no longer coherent; they were pushing apart like opposing magnets. Things just didn't fit.

As would happen many times over the ensuing years, nobody knew the pain I was in. I never let on how weird, how anxious, how utterly *different* I felt. Change had never scared me before, but this shit was different. It was an enemy I couldn't see, so I couldn't fight. The harder I searched for an explanation, the deeper I sank into confusion and then denial of my problem. I couldn't have been messed up in the head. I was the most squared-away guy I knew. Then again, that person I knew had slipped away on the big left turn a few miles back. It had to be something wrong that I could fix. Before, that had always been the way. Weak in history class—hire a tutor. A little slow running off the bike—practice my transition runs.

I'd find the problem and fix it. I was not insane. I was not insane. I was not insane. I'm not afraid of work and I'm not afraid of a fight. But show me my enemy's face.

What I needed right then was to talk, to tell my friend, any friend, myself—the whole world—just how I felt. My mind was becoming a bad neighborhood; I didn't want to go there alone. But there I sat, stranded five hundred miles from home, on a stretch of coast that had

always brought me peace and solace, hanging on to reality, bleeding
fields of pale memories, trying to spin a thread for a map home out of
the dark nothingness that comes with despair. I was in bad shape.
Alone and fucked up.

Like most people who experience psychological maladies that go
undiagnosed for a period, I was the last to admit that what I was feeling might be *in my head*. I was the sanest person around, I thought.

I knew I needed some form of help. Maybe just a few days off,
maybe sitting down with my wife and having her tell me she understood, that she might never completely *relate*, but she was in it with
me for the long run. Help would save me from going over the edge,
from feeling so confused and disoriented that I might drive my car,
and my life, right off a cliff.

I left a note for my friend, grabbed a few Power Bars and a cold
beer, and headed down the road. After a stop for gas and coffee, loud
music drowning out anything it possibly could, windows rolled
down, I pointed my car south. There were people I knew back home,
doctors and firemen and surfers and guys in wheelchairs, who had
been through some real shit. Yeah, I'd be okay. This probably was
some weird hormone deal from overtraining, or poisoning from an
abscessed tooth. Most likely hypoglycemia again.

Halfway home I started to get the "head drops," when you're so
tired you can't keep your eyes open and your head starts to bob and
drop like a spring-loaded doll head on the dash of an old car. It was
foggy outside, probably close to midnight, and I was still twenty
miles north of any city with gas and coffee and live talking people.

I pulled off the coast road onto an old farm driveway, drove over
the railroad tracks, and backed my car up next to a barbed-wire fence
tied off to a farm gate. Tucked under the overhang of a huge eucalyptus tree, I figured I was safe for a few hours and could rest my head
against the driver's window with a dirty sweatshirt for a pillow and
knock off a few zees.

Three songs and twenty minutes into my sleep, I saw the tunnel
of white light. Well I'll be darned, I thought, it's true. Heaven was calling, the light was getting brighter, the brilliance enabling me to retreat

into my own death. I knew that hope only existed when there was also doubt. But I hadn't expected to die so soon. Then somehow the doubt woke me to the terrifying sight and sound of a freight train passing by my car at eighty miles per hour, heaven's light trained on the empty tracks ahead. The subsequent rush lasted several hours, pushing me to within walking distance of my own house.

Pulling up into the driveway of my home, the house dark, the wife and kids asleep, I sat in the car and stared at the front door knowing somehow that after I passed through it, nothing would ever be the same again. I had been *affected*. Something was happening to me that I knew nothing about, except for a strange gut-level certainty that it would not go away soon. I had flashing visions of betrayal: soldiers returning from war to find their high school sweetheart married to their best friend, the family farm repossessed only hours before the back taxes were paid. But this betrayal was of my own making: My past life as a pro athlete was betraying my future before I even looked into the possibilities.

I sat in the driver's seat paralyzed until the sun came up. Then I went inside, climbed in bed with my young son, and fell asleep.

I was entering a dark place, a place of pain, renewal, despair, anger, enlightenment, depression, and maybe, if I stayed the course, understanding.

In my dreams old boxes were pried open with rusty bike rims and out flew ravens and doves and hawks and eagles. And an angel or two.

How does one describe that horrific place the mind goes when it leaves the safety of being "at peace with itself"? It is not as simple as applying a medical label; you can't just climb under the hood as you would with an old car and say, Oh yeah, it's a thrown valve, a dissociative identity disorder, a blown head gasket, an anxiety neurosis. How dare anyone try to lump the symptoms into the generic category of "mental breakdown" if they haven't been there themselves, if they haven't experienced deep mental trauma? The truth is that even brand a new Mercedes Benz will suffer small, unnoticeable breakdowns every day, same as the most mentally stable people on earth. As we do with many things, we choose to ignore it; or more likely, just don't know.

To some degree or another, everybody experiences some form of psychological difficulty during his or her life. Given the challenges of living from day to day, how could we not? Whether that spills over into the great semantic descriptive of "mental illness" should be a less urgent problem than diagnosis and treatment. Psychological challenges can range from the equivalent of a common cold to an aggressive cancer that requires institutionalization. Whoever said life was fair?

Most therapists would agree that it is always helpful to talk about psychological distress, whatever the cause. But I couldn't talk about it because I didn't think my problems were psychological. It just had to be something with the body—all those years of overtraining, all those miles of stress and strain. If I could just identify which bodily organ needed attention and take a few pills for it, or maybe some healing herbs and a few days' rest, I would be my old self again.

Six weeks later, while reading one of the hundreds of books I would devour in my search for understanding, I was struck by this quote from Viktor Frankl's *Man's Search for Meaning*. Frankl is describing how he felt when he was finally liberated after years in the Nazi concentration camps:

"I called to the Lord from my narrow prison and he answered me in the freedom of space. How long I knelt there and repeated this sentence memory can no longer recall. But I know on that day, in that hour, my new life started. Step by step I progressed, until I again became a human being."

Frankl was asking his God for a reason to go on living, a purpose to keep suffering when so many others had given up. And in his requests, he realized he still had hope, so there must be a reason, even if it wasn't obvious at the time.

I had not yet hit bottom. I was still descending into a prison hole where the creation of a new identity begins, where the past is erased so that the body's betrayal can be forgiven.

Along the way I saw no fewer than ten medical and spiritual healers: endocrinologists, urologists, acupuncturists, internists, pathologists, yoga masters, and Native American shamans. One day, after a night of being jarred awake by uncatalyzed floods of adrenaline, I decide to have an MRI to rule out an adrenal tumor. When little tumors begin to grow on any one of the organs that make up the adrenal-pituitary axis, you can have symptoms similar to what I was experiencing. Of course, you can also feel the same way from an anxiety-induced panic attack. But I hadn't gotten to that book yet.

I went to the medical building right from the beach. I was wearing my board shorts and there was sand between my toes. The lobby was filled with very sick, elderly people who were being treated for serious maladies that needed to be looked in on occasionally using magnetic resonance imaging (MRI).

All I knew was that I hadn't wanted to get out of the surf that morning, I didn't want to find out that I had an adrenal tumor, and I didn't want to put on one of those humiliating little white gowns where your bare ass announces itself to the public.

When I went into the "waiting chamber" for my turn to be strapped motionless onto a cold metal sled and conveyor-belted into a closed-in, all-telling tunnel, there was one other person in the room, a very sickly-looking older gentleman who kept eyeing me until finally he spoke.

"Happens to the best and the worst." A raspy, cough followed. "She's a scurrilous, indiscriminate disease, a real fucking bitch."

And then a young technician dressed in the ubiquitous white lab coat and wearing thick glasses that kept sliding off his pimply nose, came in and wheeled him away, leaving me to my own thoughts of mortality.

And all the people I would miss and waves I couldn't surf.

Another lab rat came for me. He asked me if I needed help climbing up onto the gurney. Three weeks before I had placed in the top ten of a professional triathlon, even though I was supposed to be retired.

I was a young man who only a few years ago was considered one of the best endurance athletes in the world. I was still tan, thin, strong, and admired. But when my head went into the MRI tunnel and the technician told me to hold very still, well, that was my bottom. I was fucked. A big part of me was dying. And I was fighting it all the way down.

What I needed to know was that it was okay to let it go, to allow that part of me to die. To give up the control I so desperately clung to; to give that control to something much greater than I.

Still, I hung on. I'd never be a great athlete again, but I could still rebel, I could still fight.

That MRI, along with every other medical test I had taken, came back negative, although I was the beneficiary of the wonderful news that my kidney held a few star-shaped stones, no doubt the result of constant dehydration from training, that would most likely pass sometime in the future.

Metaphorically, it was a little slap on the face from a girl I had offended. It wasn't the news or the sting of her fingers across my cheek, but how the jolt summoned up a needed exploration of my past and my future options: it was a shot across the bow, with another one in the hull just to keep me busy trying to stay afloat.

I just needed another war to fight, another way to express my creativeness through some essential rebellion. Stripped of my unique identity as a triathlete, I was looking at a future of normality. And it scared the hell out of me. Passing a kidney stone, I could handle. Living in a vacuum I could not.

Everyday Bad Knees

"I miss football so much—heck I even miss the interceptions."

—Archie Manning, broadcaster and
former professional football player

Athletes leave the game all the time. Maybe there's a little news clipping on page seven of the local paper noting that Bobbie Joe or Billy Ray or Tammy Sue has retired from racing or playing, both of which sound like kid's games that one doesn't so much retire from as grow out of.

The names of the stars in the limelight will change nearly every year, but other things remain the same. Hot dogs still get sold, the relish still drips on your lap. People go to work on Monday morning and push brooms, pull levers, pound computer keys, and yank chains. People still buy Gatorade to help them cut the lawn in the heat, take aspirin for sore backs, go to Super Bowl parties, and change the oil in their cars too infrequently. Kids still eat their lunch quickly at school to get a chance at being picked to play kickball. And a few parents are always late to pick up those kids from school because they got stuck in traffic or stuck on the phone or stuck in their own lives.

Some athletes are wise and pragmatic about the loss associated with leaving the game, because to them, it's not really a loss. I have a friend who was a very average runner. In his thirty-three years of average running, he completed twenty marathons, a handful of fifty-mile ultramarathons, and several thousand miles in preparation. Then one day his right knee just gave out. *No mas.* They operated to repair the torn and stretched ligaments, but like old rubber bands left out in the sun too long, they had only one more stretch left in them. You knew they'd break. He wouldn't run again.

Since I also held that activity sacred, I was afraid to ask.

"Well, are you...disappointed? I mean, how are you going to cope?"

He laughed and said, "Thirty-three years of running and cycling and football and skiing were a fine gift from that knee. Now it's time for some of those other lazy joints to pick up the slack. Something will take its place."

People wake up every day with sore knees. They wake up and use their arms to help get their legs over the edge of the bed. They groan, take a shower, feel better, walk into the kitchen to make coffee, swear when there's no milk, and somehow have a nice day through it all. It's what they do. And professional athletes, you would think, should be able to do the same, regardless of what a sore knee might mean to them. And some do, with grace and style.

In 2002, Terrell Davis retired from the NFL after seven seasons, a 1998 MVP award, and 6,413 yards rushing, the second highest total in NFL history for that time span. In 1999 he had torn the anterior cruciate ligament in his right knee and had been battling knee trouble ever since. But Davis, who had helped Denver to two Super Bowl titles, was pragmatic and mature about his situation.

"I've had all these things happen to me, and they happened for a reason," Davis told a reporter. "So if this is happening for a reason, then obviously there's something else out there better for me on the other side."

The great San Diego Padres batting champ Tony Gwynn also had a knee problem that led to profound and positive things in his life.

"It's hard to explain," he told the *San Diego Union-Tribune* soon after he retired with chronic knee problems. "I'm going through withdrawal...and I'm happy not to be playing because I don't think physically I could. But when opening day comes next season, I can't imagine how much I'm going to miss that day."

Gwynn will get over it. He's a smart guy who has a good job coaching baseball at his alma mater, San Diego State University.

People will see him standing in the dugout, pointing things out to twenty-year-old shortstops and nineteen-year-old right fielders. But they won't know how much he might be wishing to trade places with those youths, to have good knees again, to hear his name over the loudspeaker. They'll get up from their seats at Tony Gwynn Stadium on the edge of the university, walk over to buy a bag of stale peanuts, and think how wonderful it is that San Diego has a hometown hero like Gwynn and thank God they had the chance to see him play.

And when they climb into bed that night, using their arms to swing those knees up over the edge, they won't be thinking about Gwynn or Walter Payton or Roberto Clemente, they won't be thinking about their upset stomach or the meeting with the new director of finance in the morning. They won't be thinking about anything in particular except, Geez, what a great game it was tonight. And didn't Tony look good in his manager's uniform?

In one form or another, whether or not we realize it, we all get a second chance. There may exist in this world something better, something stronger than a second chance. But I can't imagine what it might be.

You would think that athletes who can choose the exact moment of their departure would have an easier time with the transition out of sport, just like choosing a home, a spouse, or the kind of car you drive—if you get to pick, chances are better you'll be satisfied.

In reality, fewer than half of all professional athletes get to choose when they'll retire, proving once again that as hard as we try to control our lives, the best we can do is put them back on track when the wheels come off.

Late in my career, when I was still racing at forty-two and forty-three years old, all anyone wanted to know was how much longer: Just how long can you keep going before your body self-destructs? I never liked the question, mostly because I could never figure out why everybody was so interested in my longevity. What is the refusal to retire but the decisive commitment to go on living anyway?

I knew my days of competing near the top were over, but I could still find my little battles to fight, even in the middle or the back of the pack. Some of the duels I fought with athletes I had never seen before and would never see again began to bother me. It's one thing to be racing for the win or a top-three finish with plenty of rewards, both material and otherwise, at stake. But a pro or even semi-pro triathlete who's struggling to swap places a zip code away from the leaders needs to examine his motivation. While I found myself accepting defeat more graciously, I also found myself reveling in the small successes that would pop up at small, out-of-the-way events.

I realized that I actually needed the competition, the thrill, the contest; it made me feel alive. Somehow, this fact troubled me. I was addicted to sport, to the hunt, the simulated kill. Sport had provided me with so much and now it wasn't letting me go. I would cross any man's fence to move up a notch or two in the standings, follow any unmarked trail. Now the exit sign was flashing in my face, neon and hideous.

I also had a growing need to be more creative, to let my "freak flag fly." I was desperately looking for more human connection, more love in my life. I was feeling the pull of the so-called *Eros* instinct, that innate impulse that attracts us to others. I had had enough of a life based on physical fitness. Sport had built me up but now it was tearing me down—*Thanatos*, the death drive, at work. I was at odds.

"The meaning of the evolution of civilization is no longer obscure to us," writes Freud in *Civilization and Its Discontents*. "It must present the struggle between Eros and Death, between the instinct of life and the instinct of destruction as it works itself out in the human species. This struggle is what all life essentially consists of."

I could detect this tension throughout my transition out of sport. I found myself starved for love on the one hand, and self-destructive on the other. I was relearning compassion for people. I began to feel emotions that had been stifled in my quest to win every race I entered. At the same time I was beating myself up. I was rife with guilt over things I wasn't even aware of and I was driving myself extremely hard at graduate school and in any activity that would put me close to the edge. I was surfing the biggest waves I could find in the winter months, reading two or three books a week, playing my guitar loud, learning how to paint, drinking too much wine, crying in secret when my teenage daughter said she hated me. *Eros* and *Thanatos* were battling for position in my new life and I was in the middle, in the vortex, getting pummeled.

I had loved my sport. It had defined me for more than half my life. It had also covered up a lot of scars. One night my wife and daughter were out and I was home with my son Dane, who was nine at the time. I was playing this really sad song I had written in a minor key, and Dane walked into the room. He just stopped and looked at me the way a nine-year-old boy looks at his dad, the way I used to look at my dad when I was nine.

"You know Dad," he began. I could tell he was trying hard to say what he needed to say as a child, but in the way an adult might attempt it. "I think I would've really liked your dad. It would be, like, super fun to say I was going surfing with my dad and my grandpa."

I smiled at him, said yeah, that would be kinda cool, huh? But he had broken through and I sat on the edge of the bed, playing my song, watching big salty tears drip all over the steel strings. Then Dane, in one of the most profound experiences I have ever had, seemed to read my mind.

"Your dad would've been proud of you. He would've kept all those race trophies and medals you gave away. He would've bragged to his friends about you. And Dad, it's okay for me to see you cry because adults need to get that sad stuff out too."

Athletes keep leaving the game. Hot dogs still get sold, the relish still drips on laps. People go to work on Monday morning and push brooms, pull levers, pound computer keys, and yank chains. Maybe there is a little news clipping on page seven of the local paper. An old-timer has died. A star has retired. You remember and a feeling washes over you. It is equal parts sadness, joy, and something altogether unnamable.

Things change and they stay the same. Kids grow up, their knees get sore, their minds a bit hardened if they're not careful, and old people die. But future stars are born every day.

When Life Decides for You

"I just decided, I'm never going to waste another day thinking about tomorrow. This is it. Today is all I have."
—Lance Armstrong, cancer survivor
and Tour de France winner

Forget everything you know, or think you know, about professional athletes. Forget that they are often envied, copied, worshipped, booed, disdained, poor-made-rich, rich-made-poor. Forget that they are both a tribute to all that the human species can become and a sobering glimpse at what our society can do as we build them up and then toss them away. Forget that they are modern day heroes and shiny Saturday morning cartoons.

Most of all, forget all that crap about sports building character and making kids strong and full of self-esteem. If you want your kids to turn out right, spend a couple of hours every day with them. And make sure you have your shit together first.

Think of athletes, for a moment, as regular men and women who followed a dream, who worked very hard, who saw an opening, and ran to it as hard and fast as their imaginations could carry them. They became special because life had given them the chance. And they took it.

Then life took it away. Only it took *everything* away, way more than it had ever given or they had ever earned. Life placed everything at their feet and then cut off their legs.

Most people can recall singular moments, when time itself stops and lets you get off for a moment and observe yourself from a distance. Everything becomes very clear and raw and present. You may repress an insight if it causes you pain, but, like a thick spring or a rebellious teen, the harder you push it down the more it wants to explode outward.

Near-death experiences can fall into this category, or the moment when a long relationship ends, the birth of a child, the death of a parent. Events like these are authentic and elemental and have the quality of bookends, forcing you to stop and see yourself in that unique way. And sometimes you witness the end of your life in one form and its beginning in another. And that experience will stay with you through every life you will ever have.

That is what happened to a few athlete friends of mine. The earthly deity they had created by virtue of fate, innate talent, and years of hard work had died. They witnessed their own deaths in slow motion.

In some ways they went to hell, felt the fire and fury, looked the devil in the eye, and said "Fuck you." They came back twisted, bloodied, but unbowed, broken in some ways, empowered and enlightened in others. They came home. And were better for their trip south.

Steve Scott was America's greatest miler. For more than twenty years he has held the record as the fastest American man over that most romantic distance in track and field competition. He earned a good living, traveled the world, and heard his name over the loudspeakers at the Olympics. The record is part of his identity, or specifically, what that record means: He has run four laps of the track faster than any man from the United States. And it brought him an enviable lifestyle.

"I had the opportunity that very few people have: to go anywhere I wanted or anywhere they have a track, which pretty much is the whole world, and to get paid to do it. I was able to live a lifestyle which very, very few people would ever have an opportunity to do, and to do it for years and years."

The mile record protected him from "the real world" of a nine-to-five job and kept the sponsors signing up years after his times had begun to slow. And even when he began to race less and dabble in sports marketing and coaching, the record made him different from the others. What it didn't do was protect him from cancer.

Steve Scott had testicular cancer, the type that spreads quickly, the type that cyclist Lance Armstrong beat, though it kills thousands every year. Scott had always been healthy and rarely injured, but with his career coming to an end there were stressors.

He had tried in vain to become the first man over forty to run under four minutes for the mile on an outdoor track. There was marital trouble, the task of raising teenagers, financial concerns. All these things Scott feels were factors in his being struck with cancer.

"There were all sorts of things going on at that time, and it started before '92, really…Obviously one was, 'What am I going to do with the rest of my life?' Number two was my earning ability was dropping, and the actual money I was bringing in was dropping. I had the cars and the kids and all this and was living beyond my means. So it's like, okay, there's this living month to month, looking at where the next money was going to come from to pay for this month's house payments. Kim [his wife] and I were going through some major difficulties in our life. We were going to see a marriage counselor. I was actually committed to ending the relationship at that point. And then we found out that she was pregnant again, so that kind of brought me back into the relationship. So—there was continual marital stress and then the running stress. I felt like because I was getting older, I had to train harder. Instead of using the skills that I had, I trained even harder than I did when I was in my twenties. Yeah, I think that those things definitely contributed to the cancer."

So Steve Scott had to decide what to do. The American record couldn't fix his marriage or his future earning power. It represented his past but did not pave his future. It wouldn't make the stress go away and it wouldn't cure his cancer. All those he had to fix on his own.

There was still one bit of information missing before he could begin to change his life. Had the cancer spread beyond his testes? Had it invaded his lymph nodes, one of the natural "filtering" components of the body? Any sign that the cancer had reached his lymph would mean that Scott would have to go through the extremely destructive process of chemotherapy.

Scott opted for the invasive operation in which samples of every major lymph node were removed from his body and inspected for cancer. And then he waited for results. Four days he waited.

What is it like to sit inside the folded petals of the poisonous flower called time? Scott lay in a hospital room with tubes running out of his nose, attended by nurses and doctors speaking a language he didn't understand but tried to interpret by tone. He had people coming to say hi, ask how he was—telling him the last time they met was on lap three of the Olympic Trials. What is it like to live in that great ghostly fog even for an hour, where the only certainty is the oppression of uncertainty?

Near the end of my career, I was given "one more chance" to be one of the best again. I was thirty-nine, maybe forty, the same age as Steve Scott when he got cancer, the same age as my dad when he died from it.

The chance came in the newly forming sub-sport of off-road triathlon: The cycling and running sections of the race were held on trails instead of pavement. This was perfect for me: I had been riding and racing mountain bikes for fun and off-season fitness long before any of the younger, faster athletes had, and technical skill is a big advantage in cycling.

All of a sudden, I was twenty-five again, racing near the front, feeling like I had staved off the inevitable decline once again, feeling like my stay of execution had come through. I trained and raced with wild abandon, rarely coming back from a ride without a new cut, scrape, or slice. My legs looked like someone had taken a weed whacker to them. I told my friend Jimmy Riccetello, who was in the same boat, relying on dirt riding and running skills to make up for advancing years, that if I didn't see blood after a race, I hadn't gone hard enough.

It was a desperate plea, one that almost put me in a wheelchair. In the fall of 1997, I careened down a long, steep hill that I had never descended before, laughing at my friends who had opted to walk down. The surface was loose ball-bearing rock, and when I hit the bottom I was going way too fast, without any control of my bike. The descent paralleled my life at that time: I had been trying to outrun something—mortality, the end of my career, the impending loss of identity—who knows?

And when my forehead hit a tree and my neck snapped back, I felt a surge of tingling flash through my body, and as I lay on the ground without feeling in my arms or legs, I saw everything go from bright white to black to the pale blue of the sky and then alternate between white and pale blue.

The terror roared in and the immutable fact was written at my feet: I had gone over the edge. Everything became very quiet, like the eerie creaking sound you hear on disaster footage after the crash, when all you see is brown dust rising up from the earth, climbing toward the heavens.

The next morning I was being rolled into a CT scan tube at the local hospital. The night before, the ER doc had failed to notice the crack in my C-6 vertebrae or the one down at T-12. In the morning, the radiologist had come in, read the X-rays, recognized my name as a former paramedic whom he had met in that same ER many years ago (a name now associated with some sort of professional sport), and kicked the machine into high gear. I suppose somebody at the hospital might have gotten a little nervous.

When they called and told me not to move, that they would send an ambulance, I felt no ill will at all. Only the dull, achy spread of deepest guilt for allowing myself to get there in the first place. All the feeling in my extremities had returned. And with it a pain of a different nature that cannot be described in words on a page.

And so, like Steve Scott, I lay motionless for several days, waiting for information that might alter the course of my life. I felt like my future was lost in time, lost *to* time.

The neurosurgeon was busy; I didn't know that my fracture was stable enough not to require an operation. Say what you want, I was a lucky son of a bitch—about as lucky as you can get in a crash like that. But there were those hours, elongated in the immaterial chains of the unknown.

Three months of immobility, another three of intense therapy, and I was tucking it away, pushing that pain into the deepest crack my mind could find. But my neck was fine, better than new.

I went in for my final evaluation with the surgeon. He reiterated how lucky I was and then, very atypical for a busy doctor, he looked out the window, adjusted the blinds of the little waiting room, and told me he hoped that I'd do something with this. He didn't have to say what "this" was.

I don't know whether I have or not. There is still time.

Steve Scott only wanted news, preferably good news.

"You asked me about an epiphany, did you?" He adjusted my question. "Was there a single moment when I knew my life would be different? Sure there was—when they told me I was okay."

Different or the same, I wanted to know.

"If they had found one single cell of cancer in my lymphs, I would've had to undergo chemotherapy."

I knew enough about that hell to know that no one comes out un-scathed. No one.

"But they didn't find anything. I knew then I was cancer-free, for the time being, and could get on with fixing my life."

That's what athletes do when they pass through those periods of intense challenge: They fix their life in some private transaction with themselves, their God, their past and present. The future is irrelevant. Athletes share an ability to focus in the moment. If they can transfer this focus to healing themselves, the future becomes only a possibility, not an item on a race schedule.

"They had to cut the cancer out of me and with it came some other things."

"Such as?"

"I've gotten much more into my faith and interest in God, and knowing that a lot of the things that I've stressed about, I could place basically upon His shoulders and just basically trust that everything's going to be okay...I've changed a lot of areas where I've gone wrong in my life."

Jim MacLaren was never a professional athlete. He may have earned a living as one of the fastest single-leg amputee runners and triath-letes ever, but his story is unique. It can never be told in written words or video clips, not with the same impact that MacLaren himself can tell the story of his rise and fall and fall and fall and rise.

It starts typically enough for a story as rife with pathos as this. Father left when he was seven years old, the oldest of four kids. Mother worked full time with Jim helping to raise his siblings, cooking meals, growing up too fast. Childhood innocence, in fact any kind of innocence, would be a luxury in his life.

Did he miss things growing up?

"Yeah, in some ways I was an adult too young because I had to be and in other ways I never grew up because I missed so much," Jim recalls. "But I knew I was smart, people told me so."

And so Jim MacLaren left home at fourteen and has been on his own ever since. That independence was important for him. It helped define him and gave him a constant target that would remain with him always, as if saying, "I can do this and I can do it all by myself," was the most important element of Jim's young life.

At twenty-two he was a graduate of Yale, where he had played football and received brilliant grades, and a budding actor with success dangling in front of him. The only thing that stood in his way was the New York City public bus that hit him square-on as he rode his motorcycle home from a job interview.

Dead on arrival at the hospital, Jim MacLaren began his long journey into the darkest of places that a human can go, to a fork that leads only in two directions: bodily death or a place where the mind is at peace with the world around it.

MacLaren doesn't recall any of that first accident. He was revived, spent eight days in a coma, and lost his left leg below the knee.

"I even underwent hypnosis to try and recall that experience," he tells me, "but I got to that intersection where the bus ran the red light and everything went black."

Before long MacLaren brought his life back into the light through his determination to be independent and to make something positive out of the tragedy. Helped by a growing interest in Eastern philosophy and spiritual practice, he graduated from the Yale School of Drama, resumed his career, and began training as a runner and triathlete. Eventually he would become the world-record holder for amputees in the marathon and a successful motivational speaker. He was regularly beating able-bodied athletes in Ironman-distance triathlons. Who needs a lower leg when you have good looks, intelligence, athletic skill, and motivation so raw and omnipotent there is not yet a word for it?

Then there was the second accident. That one was crystal-clear, slow-motion, full-framed, and very bad. Jim wasn't riding a motorcycle in the early evening traffic on a busy city street, he was competing on a bright Sunday morning in a triathlon. He was struck by a van on a course supposedly closed to traffic. His injuries were worse: a broken spinal chord at C-5, causing near-complete paralysis. The world got very, very dark again. And inside that room sat Jim MacLaren, alone, dependent.

"I thought to myself, I don't know if I can do this again."

I wanted to ask Jim what resources he drew upon. But instead I kept out of the way and let the story tell itself.

"One of my mentors told me that the hope would come back, that I had to just plant the seed and let it grow. And sometime later, I watched it."

"Watched what?"

"I was looking at the sunset and thinking, well, this is the same sun as the one that rose and set when my legs worked. And I heard myself laugh for the first time in a while and thought, that's still my voice. What's really changed anyways? I'm the same person."

Like any athlete, I wanted to know if it hurt, even if he couldn't feel it. I wanted to know if pain and suffering had become a kind of doorway for his growing insight.

"It's like this S. T. We've known a lot of shit in our lives and we can talk about it, but when I was a triathlete, just an amputee, I wasn't living it. All this stuff I knew didn't really hit me until I broke my neck. It's like what Eddy Merckx, the great Belgium cyclist used to say about pain, 'I eat it.' So behind every layer of pain there is another level and another level and another level. And at some point, pain and pleasure just become sensations. They're the same thing. So I just let the pain of being in this situation come up and find an acceptable level."

What Jim MacLaren, the former athlete, has accepted is that he will never race in any form again, not with a prosthetic leg, not in a wheel chair. His competition now takes a very noncompetitive form. MacLaren's not worried about surviving; his challenge is to play the best hand he can with the cards he's been dealt.

For an ordinary athlete that kind of transcendence is very difficult because it is external competition that defines athletes—we show the world who we are.

"That's the athlete's fire," says Jerry Sherk. "A constant opponent out there who has to be defeated so that we can show the world what is truly inside of us...There is no more 'this time,' no more coming up against a concrete opponent, no position of contender for the throne. It's rare in life when we can have such a clear task ahead of us, and a clear psychological position to do battle from."

For Jim MacLaren, though, that clarity only returned through deep exploration and acceptance. Still, after two devastating accidents, a tailspin period into a world of drugs and denial, and then a return to tell the world, I couldn't help but wonder if the psychological position from which Jim does battle is a *purgatory*, a place where he has been earthly halted to finish his training before entering some kingdom. He isn't a complete quadriplegic; he needs help with some things but lives on his own and does just fine most of the time. He knows a lot about living wounded, but still feels the draw of the topic as he works on a Ph.D. dissertation about the wounded man through time.

"The whole deal about having an incomplete injury is a mind-fuck. I can't get answers from any of the medical sources, Western, Eastern, whatever. Nobody can really tell me what to do. Only *I* can, by feeling my way from moment to moment. Some days, I have a bit of sensation in my legs and I get a glimpse of hope, but I have to paradoxically embrace it and go for it, but also deny it and be happy that I have come as far back as I have. It's hard because I want to push what I can in my constant rehab and training, but I can't get attached to it. That's the Eastern way, don't get attached to anything, the human body included."

This I had to ask Jim. If he could find out the great "why" in his tragedy, would it change anything?

"No," he says. And to make sure I understand, he says it again: "No."

The phone went quiet. Jim MacLaren had so much more to say but it was best said in the comfortable silence between us.

I said my good-byes and hung up. There was a December stillness out the window and I remembered a quote from a source that I would never find again, because to look it up would ruin the moment. I didn't want to know because that would associate it with a human source, a person. The anonymity allowed me to give it a mythical twist.

"When you die without death," it said, "no celebration of your return will ever meet your expectations."

I thought about going home. Thomas Wolfe said you can't. After two tours in Vietnam my Uncle Bill had no choice, so he said nothing and just got on with his life and buried all the shit he had seen in the deepest crack in his mind.

I know lots of athletes who have used both tactics in their return to a normal life. But the memory is always there below the surface, waiting for a time and place to poke up its head. It's not always painful; lots of people look back on their careers very fondly and are thankful to have had the chances they did. They have accepted the fact that it's over. They have no attachment to it.

Jim MacLaren didn't have a choice. Some greater force had its own idea of how he must die without death, and what the *why* in his life will be. But for MacLaren the celebration of return exceeds every expectation. Every day he rolls outside and looks at the sun.

Pulling Out

"What did those guys expect Pete Rose to do after devoting his life to nothing but baseball, get a job as a bank vice president?"

—Jim Bouton, author of *Ball Four*,
referring to criticism of Rose for selling
his sports memorabilia on television

E very athlete deals with his or her retirement in a different way, just as any human deals with loss or transition or emotional trauma: on the grounds that give them the best chance for success. Or at least they think so.

After I had exhausted all possibilities that the difficulties I faced were entirely physical, I returned to my general practitioner.

"Larry," I said, "I don't feel like I'm getting any better. And it's been six months of walking around in a type of disconnected haze."

Dr. Larry, as thoughtful and thorough a physician as you could ever want, set his chart on the table and sat down on the little roll-around stool. He pushed himself back against the wall, took off his glasses, and rubbed his eyes; he was giving me time to realize that I knew the answer to my own questions. In classic Socratic style, he was inviting me to step into the problem.

"Scott, I've run out of tests to give you. What do *you* think is wrong?"

"Well, I know now after reading all those medical texts that all thoughts and emotions have a chemical correlative—that our minds and bodies function in unison more closely than we ever thought before. I know that I put my body through about as difficult a test as one could, and I did it for over half my life. I know that there are certain activities that make the feeling better or worse; like when I'm engaged with family, friends, music, painting, or writing, or my wife and I are getting along well, it's better. When I get stressed out about the little stuff in life, like taxes and bills and just who the hell I am and what I'm going to do next...the feeling is more pervasive."

I was unraveling my problem right in front of him. We both knew it.

"Scott, let's put you through one more set of tests, a series of psycho-neurometric challenges just to rule out any real problems with mental acuity. I have a feeling you'll do fine with those and then we'll decide from there."

It was one of the smoothest, most tactful ways I've ever seen of telling someone he could use serious counseling.

Most of my life I had juggled more than one ball, always feeling that I needed to be involved in multiple projects to keep myself satisfied, if not happy. I think now it had to do with certain obsessive tendencies and a need to live life in a state of constant motion, as if every day had to be spent on the thin edge of the dime. If I slowed down or focused on only one thing or became bored or unchallenged, my coin-life might topple and take my self-motivated empire with it.

My athletic career was no different. It wasn't enough just to train and race to the best of my abilities, I had to help start and run a clothing line, give clinics, write articles, appear in training videos, consult for other manufacturers of sports products—the list goes on. In the back of my mind, I always thought that when I couldn't race as a pro anymore, when my legs finally gave way to a younger, smarter group, I'd simply do more of the non-racing stuff on the list. I'd be an athlete, in some way, forever. I was prepared, I had convinced myself; my life as a generalist would prove invaluable in my exit from sport. I could not have been more wrong.

In his book *The End of Autumn,* former NFL player and current professor of English at Oregon State University, Michael Oriard writes:

"Detachment is a key—being able to see your own football career from the outside, rather than being totally caught up in it. Football can be a seductive siren whispering in players' ears the words that can drag them to their doom. 'You're special,' it breathes. 'You're a hero;

the world admires you and wants to take care of you. Don't worry about anything; sign autographs and let people buy you drinks. You can play forever.'"

I understand that all too well now. I was well prepared and still spent four years in "adjustment," four years in a black hole of being *nobody* because I had overidentified as being *somebody* instead of just being who I was, which was *myself*.

Is it a lie we tell ourselves based on the false promises of a mixed-up society? Is it simply human nature to try and keep that ego-fulfillment going? Are we betrayed by our own trust in immortality, or at least by the strikingly painful realization that our best years are behind us and the rest of our lives will seem shallow and diminished after those days competing under a big, round July sun in front of fifty or fifty thousand people? Or is it a combination of all those, and others we haven't identified?

I do agree with Oriard that detachment is key. I was too close to the sport. The first time I began to realize this was when I read a quote I'd given in an interview. The reporter was asking how I felt about doing triathlons after all those years of competing. I told him triathlons were not what I *did* but what I *was*.

When I read that again, at first it didn't seem real. Why would I say something so bizarre and self-indicting? But on closer reflection, I knew I had said it and had meant it.

I also knew I was guilty of the indictment. I had taken the sport in and made it my primary source of socialization, identity, fulfillment, and release. I had a great wife and two incredible young kids. The kids were the love of my life. But at the time, the sport gave me things that they were not able to yet.

The sport allowed me to explore, to search, to travel, to suffer, to relate, to dig into my past, to cover up my past, to pretend to be a superstar or a simple, humble kid who got lucky. I was like an Etch A Sketch on which I could draw my self-image and show it to the world if I felt like it—or just turn it over and shake away the mistakes.

The luckiest ones have someone who can understand, to listen to you speak in tongues they might not know the exact translation to but could ascertain the meaning by your tone, your eyes, and the shape of your heart that rests in your hands.

A focused, traveling, competing athlete has difficulty nurturing a relationship that can provide that.

Now, if you are thinking how difficult this type of transition must be on a marriage, you would be quite correct. While the major leagues such as baseball, basketball, football, and hockey do not record such data—and if the retired players associations do, they are not telling—I have it from reliable sources that the divorce rate for pro athletes post-retirement is between 60% and 70% within the first two years. In my own athletic circles, at least seven of my closer friends divorced within a few years after they retired.

When my wife of nearly twenty-five years and I found ourselves in marital trouble after I relinquished the title "professional athlete," we both thought about splitting up; the work needed to figure out what was going on seemed overwhelming.

It makes perfect sense that this would happen. Star athletes have a persona, an image, a certain "shtick" that surrounds them. Sometimes the athlete creates it for competitive reasons (e.g., a boxer's rowdy prefight weigh-in); other times the media create it to make a player more interesting. In any case, the image is not always true to the athlete's self, although he or she may come to maintain it, if not believe it, over time.

When athletes form relationships, they are often based on the fabricated personality. The non-player may not have known the player before he or she was an athlete. And when the player retires, the persona is stripped away, sometimes slowly, if the player hangs on, other times suddenly.

Retiring players often begin a process of discovery and an effort to return to their true selves. The mate is now forced to reflect on exactly who it is he or she is living with. Rarely does a person retiring from a lifetime of high-level sport *not* change in some profound way. The mate can either accept the change—maybe he or she adapts and changes too—or deny it.

The evidence, anecdotal as it may be, suggests that the second response is more common. In all honesty, it's hard on both parties. I wanted someone to go through it with. But as we've said, if you haven't been there, how can you relate? And who was I to ask such a thing of *anybody*, regardless of the connection?

I simultaneously felt disappointed with Virginia for not being more supportive in my time of need and disappointed with myself for expecting so much. What I was asking requires incredible love, compassion, and commitment, more than many relationships can bear. I doubt I could have served the role had the positions been reversed.

As the years unfolded, I came to realize that she was just reacting to my metamorphosis. And it scared her. We had known each other for ten years before I ever made any real money at the sport. We had grown up as a young couple struggling to get ahead, enjoying the simple things in a simple life. Now the challenge was to return to a life like that and for both parties to accept it and accept each other in their new roles. It was a decision we had to make, a choice of some consequence since we had two kids and had spent most of our lives together. We pushed through it and, though no one can call us Ozzie and Harriet, I have more admiration and respect for Virginia because of the challenge.

I have learned that the root of many of these problems is a distorted sense of ego. Not an enlarged ego, but a distorted one. I knew then, and I know better now, that my life in sport was at times real and at times a projected silver-screen image. Things got confused when I accepted that image and ran with it unchecked. I became a parody of myself; the truth was behind it but a false perception was in front of it.

We laugh about it now, but when Jim Curl, the cofounder of the first series of national-level triathlon events, consulted me about the proper balance of distances among the three sports, I convinced him to make the run relatively longer than the rest. Why? Why else? I was a runner. For two years, thousands of participants in his series ran an extra 5K because I had let my love of control, my ego, overcome my sense of fairness. Actually, I don't think it was so much selfish as it was rebellious.

To all those who suffered that extra twenty minutes in those early races, I apologize here and now.

Many years later when my life unraveled in the face of my impending exit from sport, I contacted my old friend Steve Estes. Steve had been my rowing coach in college one year and had gone on to distinguish himself in academia; at the time he was acting as chairman of the physical education and kinesiology department of a small East Coast college. Not bad for a former national-class athlete who still doesn't have a clue what he wants to be when he grows up.

I'm sure my effort to track him down had a lot to do with my self-prescribed healing method: to seek out and find other retired athletes. What did they experience? Had they felt any of the strange emotions that I did? How did they cope with the difficulties in transition? What tools did they rely upon to move through the pain?

When I first met Jerry Sherk, the former Cleveland Brown, I asked him if there was some sort of book or manual I could read that would help me. Well, Jerry laughed and no, sorry, nothing like that existed that he knew of. I was disappointed, but Jerry gave me a greater challenge.

"You don't need a manual. You need to open your mind to the possibilities. Let go and think."

Then he told me to read the philosophers Nietzsche and Heidegger, the mythologist Joseph Campbell, social theorists like Mead and Cooley, and C. Wright Mills. That would be a good start, he said. They won't give you answers but they will remind you that you are not alone.

One day I received a long letter from Steve Estes. He was writing from Scotland, it was late at night there, and he had just returned from a pub. He apologized for taking so long to get back to me and then proceeded to take his place in line with a handful of former athletes who would put me back on track, help me find a better, truer self, and challenge me to find that which I sought—answers to all these question about life after sport.

It wasn't the exact words of advice that my old friend and coach offered, but the fact that he offered them at all. As I noted earlier, what athletes miss are the other athletes. The other athletes accept each other for whoever they are at the moment—the cocky kid who scored the game-winning basket or the lonely man-child who confides that he misses home.

One thing you learn to do well as a professional athlete playing on a team is to empathize with the other players. You learn this not because you are taught by the coaches, to make you a better-functioning unit, but because you too need that support. It is a wonderfully soft thing in a very hard world.

And when you are pulled from that world, the first call you make is not to your parents or your agent or your spouse—it is to one of your old teammates, because they have *earned* that call.

Most people had no idea what I was going through. That was fine with me. I didn't want sympathy—I knew I had to go through this on my own. But now, as a writer, I wish I had been writing more from that "place" that one inhabits in moments of despair, love, great joy, and terrible angst—the true moments when human emotion has no barriers and flows with clarity and beauty. Even in the darkest of life's moments, there is humor, compassion, irony, and vibrancy. At such moments we are connected to our maker, to the earth, to every other living creature. This gives them a certain beauty.

I had shared my feelings with a few close friends and they were my life rafts, because somehow they knew what to say, when to make me laugh, when to tell me to get my shit together, and they always told the truth.

One of my friends is a firefighter/paramedic with the appropriate name of Jimmy Black. For a period, he would call me up every other day and just ask, "Howz your head?" But Jimmy is a healer, that's his genius. In the summer of 2002, when I had half of my nose cut off due to skin cancer, he came over right after I returned from the hospital and asked to see my scar.

"Dude, that is so gnarly. It's still oozing out of the suture lines."

"Hey you want to see the picture before they spliced a piece on?"

"Oh, yeah. Check it out. You look like a Halloween mask. Hey, what did they do? Take a piece of your ass and paste it on? Are you going to have butt hair growing out of your nose?"

"Naw, man, the guy was a fucking genius, just sculpted the edges into a new tip. It could've been a lot worse."

"Yeah, it can always be worse. We're so lucky. Check it out—we're healthy, got good families that act like they love us, probably do at times. We don't work shitty office jobs and we still rip on a short board."

"I hear you. I really don't care about the nose. It's only body parts. It won't affect my cutback or my tube rides. It's too bad they didn't chop half of your schnoz. That thing could use some trimming."

"My time will come—the sins of our youth and all that shit. You better come over and cheer my ass up when I'm all bust up."

"Damn straight. If I know the doc or she is some kind of sports fan, I'm scrubbing up and going into the OR, see if I can still start an IV on your pencil wrist with one hand like I used to."

"Screw that. You'll just make sure I'm not as pretty as you, try and keep all the chicks for yourself."

"What are friends for?"

But I didn't have to ask and Jimmy, he already knew too well.

It's easy to laugh at loss years after it's passed and you've survived it. But it takes true courage to take it in the moment and bend it and shape it until it turns into an opportunity for growth, love, compassion, and sometimes, if necessary, more loss. It takes friends like Jimmy Black to know when to make you laugh, when to let you cry, and when to just sit there and play the guitar while you stare off into space, trying to find your place in the world somewhere between the cradle and the grave, between the bliss of childhood and the tumult of teen years, between the responsibility that comes with survival and the responsibility that comes with wisdom. It takes people like Jimmy Black and Jimmy Riccetello, athletes every one of them but with hearts as big as Saint Bernards, to be there when you fall, to say nothing for as long as it takes, and then to stop and say, "You ain't goin' down, okay? Bunch of geeks out there love your ass. Probably God too. Now, listen to this riff."

Coping and Support

*"I haven't had any opportunistic infections. I'm just doing
real, real well."*

—Greg Louganis, Olympic gold
medalist, at age forty-two

I had his home phone number. A mutual friend set it up. The
"world's fastest human" had agreed to talk to me, to tell me
about his successes, his frustrations, his bitterness, and his hope.
Then he died.

Bob Hayes, gold medal winner in the 1964 Olympics with a world
record—tying 10.06 seconds for the one hundred meters, Bob Hayes,
the NFL star receiver with the Dallas Cowboys who still holds a
record for seventy-one touchdowns scored in his ten seasons with the
team, and Bob Hayes, the man whose life after sport was a series of
tragedies he could not outrun.

In 1979 Hayes was arrested and charged with distribution of cocaine; he eventually served ten months of a five-year prison term. He
long struggled with alcoholism and was denied entry into the NFL
Hall of Fame because of his prison time.

Jerry Jones, the owner of the Cowboys, said upon hearing of
Hayes's death of prostate cancer in 2002, "I've never seen a professional athlete who was more universally loved—by all his teammates—than Bob Hayes." And Jones has seen many.

No one can say for sure why Hayes sold cocaine, why he drank.
Lots of ex-pros abuse alcohol or drugs while they are in the pain and tumult of transition. It's a common method of coping with the problems

that rear their head, the things they feel or don't feel. Alcohol and drugs
help them forget for a while and let them feel things they may have forgotten how to feel. In a study done on forty-eight retired athletes out of
the University of Western Australia, researchers found that alcohol and
drug use was listed in the top fifteen of coping mechanisms, right
below "denial" and right above "turning to religion."

Nobody is saying that it's good to use alcohol or that you must
"turn to religion" to find yourself after sport. In the case of substance
abuse, it can delay the return to normalcy and contentment; it can
only complicate the issues. But denial in some form, at some point, is
a near-universal response to loss. And the only way through denial is
to go *through it.*

But maybe you still have a hard time offering compassion to these
retired athletes. Like others, you reserve it for people who need it
most—the homeless, the sick, the old and forgotten, yourself. Yeah,
maybe you too know what it's like. "How can it be?" you may have
asked yourself. "He was right here yesterday." Or, "How could I lose
that job? I worked so hard." Or, "That was my dream house, I
would've died there." And in the beginning you denied that it was
gone. You denied yourself the pain.

Maybe you are one of the growing number of sports fans who just
don't know what to feel about the players or the teams these days.
They don't seem loyal to you. What do you owe them? Every day you
read in the paper about an athlete who has gotten himself into trouble. (Of course, the papers rarely follow up on the results; it's just not
that newsworthy when someone is acquitted, or a story turns out to
be a hoax.)

On September 21, 2002, I read a short clip off the wire services that
a woman had accused baseball Hall of Famer Kirby Puckett of sexually
assaulting her in the bathroom of an Eden Prairie, Minnesota restaurant. Later I found out that Puckett had been charged with a felony
count of false imprisonment and a gross misdemeanor count of crimi-
nal sexual conduct. One of Puckett's attorneys said, "The only reason
Kirby Puckett was charged today is because he is a famous person. If
this were anybody else, this case would have never seen the light of

day." As a student of the sociology of sport, I was interested. As a human being, I had to think it a tragedy, regardless of truth or blame.

The same day I read that three-time Wimbledon champion Boris Becker was scheduled to go on trial in October in Munich on tax evasion charges. The news report said there was a lawsuit seeking $1.47 million in unpaid taxes. I wonder how it turned out. A week later I saw a friend's name in the same "sports and courts" section of paper. He had been charged with a serious crime. How do you deal with that? He's not a close friend so I didn't call, but still I felt odd for not doing *anything*. It makes you wonder how people would react to seeing your name in the paper with words like "alleged" and "bail" in the article.

It is a difficult situation to label or choose sides in. The best we can do is understand, learn, and assist. There are no hand-washing political sound bites—no "just say no" or "they made the decision for us." When an individual is deliberately coddled and sheltered from the distracting obligations of life, he or she may not develop the same sense of responsibility for one's actions. Many professional athletes have to go back and pick up necessary social skills when they lose the protective bubble of sport—and just as they are trying to cope with the loss of everything that was in the bubble with them.

Denial is natural. Getting knocked down hurts. Do you think Michael Jordan likes to acknowledge that he paid a woman $250,000 a decade ago? No way. Jordan is first and last a basketball player. Somewhere along the way he might have made an error in judgment—he became human. He had to admit that error. Jordan now charges that the woman wants an additional $5 million to remain quiet about their relationship. It makes you wonder where the error in human judgment lies. It makes you realize that we all make mistakes but only a few of us see them played out on page one of the sports section with lots of zeros in the details.

It is no wonder that some athletes resist the return to normalcy. There is too much duplicity, too many gray areas. People want to remember you as an athlete. You have to convince them that you can do something else, be somebody else. Sometimes you feel like a child asking for approval. But you are a grown man or woman trying to move forward.

I remember Linda Buchanan, one of the best female triathletes in the world at one time, complaining about her relatives. Linda had retired and gone on to graduate school and to a successful career in upper management with a sports product company, as well as a part-time job coaching water polo. But it seems that some of her extended family couldn't get over the fact that she wasn't a big sports star any more.

That's a tough situation. I'm sure she was polite and tactful, but in a way it requires more coping skills than many athletes have.

When I finally tired of answering questions about my next race or how my training was going, even years after I left the pro ranks, I wasn't so cordial. I would push the questions away, saying, "I don't know. I don't live in that world anymore."

But for many of them, I did. My old identity was changing with each day of my acceptance. Now if only the others could accept the fact that athletes change.

The follow-up to denial is usually depression or anger. It depends on the person. I never really felt the anger. Or if I did, it presented itself as guilt and I was harder on myself than I had been before.

Everybody gets depressed at certain periods in life. Some just hide it better than others. Heck, nobody likes to listen to someone complain. We are a nation of independent survivors—always have been. Depression just gets in the way.

Last December I stopped during a long bike ride to talk to a man standing next to a freeway on-ramp. He was holding a sign that said, "Why lie? I need a beer." I told him he had panache, asking for money that way, and gave him $10—$5 for a six-pack, $5 for his creativity. He told me he only had one rain poncho and he wouldn't sell it for $10. That would be too big a loss. Funny thing, he didn't look depressed.

Coping with loss is like those candied apples. Tap it in the right spot and it falls apart in sections.

Much has improved in recent years for retiring pro athletes, especially those who play the major team sports, basketball, baseball, football, and hockey. Gone are the days when a player like star receiver and Super Bowl winner Don Maynard had to work in the off-season as a plumber to make a living. The combined average annual salary in these leagues is close to a million dollars. Now, that's the average, not the minimum, but even if a player only plays for four or five years at $500,000 annually, that money, invested safely and combined with a modest lifestyle—two things not always assured—should provide a financial cushion. At least that's one less thing they have to worry about.

My research has shown that many of the players who retired before there was the huge money in the leagues seem to have had easier transitions, psychologically, from pro sports to the real world—although I'm sure a lot them could use a piece of those twenty-first-century multi-million-dollar contracts. For them, however, there is assistance from their old leagues.

"We gave away close to $5 million last year to ex-players in need, all through the PAT," says Dee Becker, an executive with the National Football League Players Association. PAT stands for Player's Assistance Trust. I was amazed.

"You gave away $5 million?" I asked incredulously, forgetting for a moment that most of the players who retired ten or fifteen years ago probably had done so without a large financial portfolio. They retired with the same sore backs and torn-up knees as the guys who are retiring now, but with substantially fewer zeros in their checking account.

"In 1984, the NFL Retired Players Association had 300 members," Becker added, "Today [early 2003] we have 3,500 members in thirty-one different chapters around the country."

This was encouraging, although the rise in membership over the years was not surprising. What is more encouraging is that the trend within the league, within the Players Association, and among the individual teams has been to urge players to take part in the programs offered while they are still playing, not after they retire and suddenly realize they have to deal with this thing called life.

Jerry Sherk, who heads up the San Diego Chapter of the NFL Retired Players Association, finds a few things interesting.

"Often we don't see a player come to a meeting or join the group until four or five years have passed since they left the game. Then they come around and start asking about services or just talking to others about their experiences after they quit."

One might surmise that a player has to separate himself from the game for a while, to find his new identity, before returning to the fold. Or maybe they try for years to make it on their own and in the end realize that talking about the game and the years after the game with others who can truly relate is the best way of healing.

The question of responsibility remains: Who should carry these former stars when they don't shine anymore? Is it the league, which runs a multi-million-dollar business whose main products are the bodies and minds of the players? Is it the Players Association, the union if you will, that is supposed to look after the players' best interest? Is it the individual teams, who know that each player is only valuable when he performs for the paying crowd? Or is it the players themselves who need to shoulder the task of dealing with their lives, both before and after they retire?

"We are finally seeing some cooperation between all parties," says Dr. Jeff Erkenbeck, a psychologist and former consultant to the NFL Player Development. "There are some excellent programs in place for active players to develop skills that will help them beyond the game. What needs to happen is for more players to take advantage of them."

No one can say for sure why the NFL Players Association has begun a push to prepare their players for life after football. After all, when it comes right down to it, when you put the NFL itself, or the individually owned teams up against the players unions, it becomes a classic management-labor situation. But it must be a win-win at the same time.

All players will someday retire, whether or not they prepare themselves for that day. To offer them information, choices, training, and encouragement is a must.

"The key," says Dr. Erkenbeck, "is to get them involved early on in their career. They can choose from programs in corporate development, youth coaching, media training—there's lots of good stuff now."

Some players, though, think it's too little, too late. One ex-player who requested anonymity said, "It doesn't look good on the league when you have a whole bunch of ex-players who are dying young, getting in trouble with the law, or basically leading shitty lives after football. Whatever they are doing they ought to double."

No one can blame an ex-player who feels like he was used as a "piece of meat" if he is dealing with the consequences. Even the fans who are inclined to believe that ex-players can buy happiness with all that money they were paid need to reevaluate their position.

Nevertheless, for whatever reason, there is a growing movement toward supporting the players, based on foresight, vision, and large numbers of ex-players returning to the game to help run these programs. For instance, Gene Upshaw, the director of the NFL Players Association since 1983, was a player in the NFL with the Raiders. Ron George, director of player development for the San Diego Chargers, was a linebacker in the NFL for eight years, playing for the Atlanta Falcons and then Kansas City.

In fact, the establishment of a specific "Player Development" position within each team in the league may not be mandated but it is "strongly encouraged," as one official put it. Of course, some teams place more emphasis on the position than others. Ron George takes his job with the Chargers very seriously. Most people like George do. They know what it's like because they've been there.

"There are lots of success stories of retired players who went on to live successful, well-adjusted lives," says George, "but they aren't as well publicized or as interesting to the public as the stories of those who have fallen on their face."

I would agree and add myself to the list of those who are guilty of finding pathos better copy than uneventful transition. But those are the people who need the help. The ones that struggle and suffer need their stories told. Exposing a problem is the first step in fixing it.

Before every team had a person like Ron George, the important duties of preparing athletes for a life after sport were either ignored or given little import. I was told by one source that before George, the person fulfilling the duties of "counseling and guiding" the active

Chargers players was "some guy who was the director of security or something."

I don't know many security guards trained in counseling.

"You have to look at this as a business model," says Dr. Joel Fish of the Center for Sports Psychology in Philadelphia. "There is a relationship between an employer and an employee. Certain resources should be offered. There would be a limit to how long certain services would be offered to an ex-player, but all that would be negotiated and known early in their career."

And to some extent, that's what the major leagues and their related associations of retired players have done—look at how they can help, but also keep an eye on the business aspect of things.

In baseball, there is the Major League Baseball Players Alumni Association. Their focus is on providing income and publicity opportunities for ex-players through Legends-style events, speaking engagements, and the like. There is also the Baseball Assistance Team (B.A.T.), but it isn't affiliated with the league or the Players Union in any way.

"There are no dues or membership," says Jim Martin, the executive director. "Our mission is to help members of the 'baseball family' from all ages, the minor leagues to the old Negro Leagues. The only criteria is need."

Started in 1986 through funding from an insurance company, catalyzed by then Commissioner of Baseball Peter Ueberroth, the organization has raised and distributed over $10 million for needy players.

And if for a moment you think that term might be an oxymoron, think again. Thousands of men have made it to the pros in baseball. A very, very small percentage have received the huge compensation packages that make the sports pages. The destitute players who gave so much to the game and had life turn on them after they left, those are the guys who deserve a piece of the Major League Baseball pie, which is worth many times that $10 million figure.

Triathlon doesn't have a players' assistance team; most individual sports don't even have an 800 number. What they have is each other. And when no one is around you, sometimes anybody with an ear will do.

In one of the last years I was competing seriously, I found myself alone at a hotel the night after the race. I couldn't get out until the next day, so I wandered down to the restaurant for a salad and my requisite two glasses of passable cabernet as prescribed by Dr. Jimmy Black. When the waitress, a local gal named Marge with that look that says, "I'm here because I didn't get the big part in that movie I auditioned for twenty years ago," asked me how many were in my party, I had to think for a minute. "One," I told her, "I'm here by myself because I'm a loner, no friends, washed up, over the hill, barely made the top five today."

Marge looked at me and shook her head as if to say, "Don't dump your shit on me honey, I got my own to swim through." After the first glass of wine I noticed a wedding party being held outside on the expansive lawn inside an even more expansive tent. After the second glass I asked Marge if she knew the wedding party. Sure she did, it was a local family, the daughter of a guy who rode his mountain bike in the hills behind the hotel. This was getting interesting. I paid Marge and walked out to the tent for a better view.

There is something inside of us all, some Eddie Haskell personality trait, that dares the other parts of our psyche to push the envelope from time to time for no other reason than to see how far it will stretch. That something nudged me on the shoulder and asked me to dance, or maybe it was the other way around, but twenty minutes and two beers later I was on the dance floor with the bride, wearing shorts and wishing her well. And when I finally sat down and saw one hundred pairs of eyes on me, a man close to my own age sat down next to me and asked if I was having a good time.

"Sure, this is a great wedding, isn't it," I shucked and jived. "Don't they make a great couple?"

"They better because I'm the father of the bride and the man footing the bill for this whole thing."

"I'm sorry, I was just lonely and one thing led to another and I'll pay for my drinks and..."

"Listen Tinley..."

"You, uh...*know* me?"

"I've lived here in this town all my life. Used to come out here and watch you and Molina race this course every year. You inspired me to compete a few times. You are as welcome at this wedding as anybody. My daughter and her groom grew up with stories about you triathletes. I'm glad you're here."

I left the tent, stunned, not knowing what to do or how to feel. The best I could do was to return to my room, pick up my fourth-place trophy, take it back to the tent, and add it to the pile of gifts for the lucky couple. And walk off into the night, thankful for people like that.

Part Four

▼ ▼ ▼

ASHES TO ASHES: GOLD TO GOAL

Where Do They Go?

We shall not cease from exploration
And the end of all our exploring
Will be to arrive where we started
And know the place for the first time.

—T. S. Eliot

This is the question that is first asked of a retiring athlete. This is the question that people will ask out of politeness, or for lack of any other words, or in case the athlete might actually want to talk about it. Sometimes it's even asked out of some deeper concern for the athlete's well-being, which is never in the same way as a reporter looking for a sound bite.

The question is: What next?

Two simple words that carry the weight of the past into the future on the shoulders of some ambiguous present. Some athletes know. The lucky ones have thought about it, given it serious consideration while they were playing. Rarer still are the ones who have always known.

Eric Heiden knew. Cal Ripken, Jr. knew. And in their knowing, however it was derived, lies the seemingly pain-free transition out of sport.

Many have thought a bit about what they would do—work on an investment project they bought into, do TV commentary, work in marketing for an old sponsor. That seems natural. Maybe they fully understood that they were a type of glorified sandwich board to advertise the company's product and could easily move into the role of passing out the cash instead of asking for it.

The unlucky ones figure they have enough money to be whoever they want. If they lacked an identity or became lonely, well, everything is for sale, right? Just open a restaurant with their name on it and people will flock in with the hopes that the star might be sitting there at the bar, holding court, buying drinks, regaling the crowd with tales of his youth, *your* youth.

But the fact is, fewer than 25% of new restaurants last a year in business. Restaurants, fancy-footwork investment schemes, fancier cars—they're just Band-Aids really. If you work at it, you end up where you belong—where we all belong—in a place that makes you happy, where you feel fulfilled and needed. And that is something that money cannot buy.

When I asked athletes who have been retired for a long time what the biggest difference is between them and the athletes coming out now, three quarters of them suggested that the younger athletes had been affected, almost always adversely, by the huge increases in money.

Don Maynard, NFL Hall of Famer, member of the 1969 Super Bowl-winning New York Jets, and one of the great wide receivers of the late '60s, said that he couldn't afford to be "just one of the best players in the league."

"I got out of college," he remembers, "and I was making $4,600 a year. Then I signed with the Giants in 1958 for $7,500. Now, you couldn't live off of that, so in the off-season I was making $8,500 as a plumber."

"A plumber?" I asked him.

"Yep. It takes five years to become a licensed plumber. That's why I think of it more as an engineering degree."

That type of preparation, one can imagine, was invaluable when the athlete's career is over, mostly because sport was never a lifetime career. It was something that a player did for a limited number of years. He made some money, hopefully enjoyed his time, and after a while went back to whatever he was doing before the *opportunity* to play in the pros came along.

In a way, retiring from sport with lots of money in the bank is a curse. You don't *have* to work. Which means you can lie in bed all day, never lift a finger, never answer the phone, just stare at the wall and wonder who the hell you are.

I retired with only a few years' worth of what I called "retooling" money, just enough to allow about two years of schooling to prepare for something else. But when it all hit me and I went into that void between lives, I had a few of those days, just lying in bed, staring at the wall. Actually, if I added up all the hours in my years in transition, it was more like a few months.

Those were hellish hours, crumpled up in some little corner of the world that I thought would give me solace, would give me the time and space I needed to figure out who I had been, so that I could move onto what I really was. In between was the vacuous nightmare of nothing, a bridge without a beginning or an end.

Despite the great number of athletes that go through this period, it seems that few, myself included, can accurately describe what it feels like.

In his book *You Cannot Be Serious*, the tennis legend John McEnroe writes, "But once your career is over you're in a funny place if you've done reasonably well as a professional athlete, namely: Where do you go from here?"

Now, McEnroe is a smart man, maybe one of the more intelligent professional athletes I've seen over the years. To watch him do TV commentary now, he appears to be an entirely different person than when he was a young, sometimes angry player. "I've given a lot of hard thought to who I was," he continues in his book, "who I am, and who I want to become."

Some of the change could be attributed to a simple maturation process: "I've done a lot of growing up over the past quarter century. On the other hand, like most people...I'm still a work in progress."

Aren't we all John?

Still, not everyone devotes the "hard thought" to find out who he or she is. Quite often it takes someone else to point that out. Many of the people around me at the time I retired were very stable, loving individuals. As hard as it was for me to have an honest, open con- versation with myself, it was even harder for me to speak with them about it. As Steve Estes had told me, they hadn't *earned* the conver- sation. I know that sounds egotistical, but unless you have suffered similar emotional trauma, it is very difficult to relate.

Do you ever wonder about the past lives of psychologists, psy- chiatrists, and counselors? Most of them can relate to their patients in some way because they have "been there," they've walked a mile in those messed up shoes. They know.

I once took this up with a friend of mine, a psychiatrist I had be- friended because he was a good man, because he could help me, be- cause I trusted him, because I got the sense he had been through some shit himself.

"What is the percentage of individuals in your profession who have experienced some form of emotional trauma in their past?" I asked him.

"Are you kidding?" he said. "That's why we get into this gig: We know it, we have the capacity to be good at it, and it's an ongoing form of healing for us to help others."

For the retiring athlete who sticks around his or her sport, work- ing as a coach, an administrator, a TV analyst, or in a marketing or sales job, it can't be much different.

Sport is what athletes know, it's what they have been trained to do. Many want and *need* to stay around their sport in some way: some because they enjoy it, some because they feel good giving back, and some because they don't really have a lot of other options.

I know a couple of world-class ice skaters who literally bank on a strong performance in the World Championships or the Olympics. If they slip, it's back to the day job. If they are lucky and skate well, a few temporary endorsements followed by a job as a coach at some club, assuming they want to remain close to the sport. Once in a great while someone will rise out of the fringe sports and become a house- hold name. Frank Shorter won the gold medal at the 1972 Olympic marathon in Munich, effectively launching the running boom in the process. The skater Dorothy Hamill transferred her perky nose and picture-bob haircut from a quadrennial Olympic broadcast to the professionally produced *Champions on Ice* show, coming to an arena near you. World Surfing Champion Kelly Slater appeared as a cover boy for mainstream magazines, produced a passable CD with fellow surfer musicians, and dated Pamela Anderson Lee of *Baywatch*—hey, whatever is takes. The bottom line is that they were all the best at what they did, they were given the breaks, and they ran with them.

With money, though, the question of how much is always relative. Often it has more to do with self-esteem than with paying the rent. Some of the better-paid athletes realize that it would be difficult even to spend the amounts they are compensated. The sum their agents negotiate for is often a symbol of how much the team values them, and whether the team owners feel confident that the fans will pay for that seven-figure salary each year. Seven-figure salaries for pro athletes are a truly idiosyncratic twist to modern capitalism. The layman's discussion will often center on whether or not the athlete *deserves* that amount. But that's not the issue. Fair market value is established by what a willing buyer will pay a willing seller.

As with other high-profile entertainers, a high market value is established for top athletes. Why? Sport is the last major form of entertainment in our society in which the ending is not predictable. Most everything else, from cinema to symphony, from screenplay to surrealistic art, has taken on a formulaic feel. The commodification of what was once labeled sacred—the arts—has blurred the lines of pleasure. Sport resembles art in the purity of the performance and in the creativity and beauty of the acts. It is entertainment because people want to see those acts performed live, they want to say that they saw the last game that Gretzky ever played, to tell their grandchildren about it, to relish their association with a historic figure.

Many highly paid athletes become accustomed to a certain income and the status that comes with it. When the income stream dries up, there is rarely an automatic scaling-back in lifestyle. Money can be a curse. It's the adage, The more you have, the more you need.

If you don't have much, what you need is a job to pay the bills. A job gives you purpose, direction, and identity, the very things that are often absent when a wealthy athlete retires. The first job may not be the right one, but it's like lighter fluid on the coals—it moves the process in the right direction.

The "what next" question recurs. How are athletes to consider it in the context of where they have been, where they think they want to go, and ultimately, where they need to be. What do you do after you did what you were born to do? What kind of job follows destiny?

For all those who feel lucky to segue immediately into a job associated with their sport, there are those who need a separation before returning to the sport that was their life for so many years.

Rick Sutcliffe, Cy Young Award winner and potential Hall of Fame member, was not one to re-embrace baseball instantly upon retirement. He recalls:

"Well, the funny part was, I said, I'm like a lot of people—I'm getting so far away from this game—I'm not coaching. You'll never see me again! I'm going to go fishing, I'm hunting, I'm golfing. And I did that. I was pretty much 'America's Guest' in 1995. All the tournaments you get invited to, one a day—fly to Hawaii, stay here, do this—I mean it's just unbelievable, the opportunities. And after about three months of doing that, I was sick of it. And at the end of that year I looked back and I had accomplished nothing, I had bettered myself in no way whatsoever. There had to be a reason to get up in the morning other than just making playtime."

Years later, Sutcliffe has made his peace with baseball, which is to say he has made his peace with his past. Between coaching and television work, he is involved in the game from a different perspective, one that has little to do with sore arms and more to do with giving back. Rick Sutcliffe has accepted his new role and his new life. Now he is whole again—inside a new uniform.

It can help tremendously if an athlete feels that he or she has accomplished something in sport. If you are forced out or retire before you are ready, the stage is set for a more traumatic retirement. But if you can look back and say, "Well, I did something," it makes the transition easier.

"There is a bridge that must be crossed by all who leave the game or have the game taken from them," writes Bill Lyon in *When the Clock Runs Out*. "When you get to the other side, you meet the other you."

The key to making it across seems to be perseverance and a deep conviction that no matter how difficult the transition, you will eventually make it to the other side and meet the "other you," who quite often is a truer you. If you turn back, it must be for the right reasons. If not, it will only make the journey longer and more difficult.

Another question faced by the retiring athlete, or anybody in transition, is: What *can* I do?

The answer, again, is infinitely duplicitous. You can do whatever you put your mind to, but only what you are able. It depends on your resources, including patience, work ethic, abilities, and bank account level.

If you want to be the president of your own company, and you have the financial means to do it, you can simply buy a little outfit and name yourself president. If you want to be a coach, well, it may take a while to find a head coaching job on a major league baseball team, but I know of plenty of little league teams and YMCAs that would be more than happy to give a former pro player a group of kids to handle. Tim Flannery did it. Let go from his position with the San Diego Padres with a year left on his contract, he would often say that he was the highest paid coach in little league baseball.

It can take a while to retool yourself, especially if you haven't worked at a skill while you were playing. Or even if you have.

I asked Don Maynard if his off-season work, first as a licensed plumber and then as a financial planner, helped his transition.

Well, I continued to do those things," he remembers, "but after seventeen years of playing pro ball, I found that I was seventeen years behind all of my buddies who graduated out of college and went straight to work. I was going to coach and teach and all that, so I got out and now all my buddies are head coaches and principals and superintendents, and they're making sixty-five, eighty-five, a hundred thousand dollars a year, and I'm back here starting life over at the bottom of the ladder. And, ah, it's been a tough row to hoe."

Patience and hard work have made Don Maynard a successful and content businessman. But he will always be an ex-player.

Sometimes when players retire and look to the things that made them feel whole and content while playing, they realize that much of it had to do with physical activity. And now the body is worn out. It can't run eighty miles a week, it can't log three or four hours a day on the ice or two hours in the pool. Players must then turn inward and find their purpose and their passion through a non-physical connection to the world. Those who are permanently injured are faced with this daunting question every day for the rest of their lives: What can I do now that will give my life meaning, but won't require me to be a superior physical being?

For others who retire with only a few aches and pains, the question returns to: What can I put my mind to? For NFL greats Paul Hornung and Herschel Walker, the business environment presented a new arena for challenge and success. Today Hornung is the owner of a Louisville-based real estate and cooking oil company.

Walker, a terribly nice man who once beat me in a semi-final tennis match at the annual Super Stars Competition (a loss my tennis buddies still like to bring up), has also done well in several entrepreneurial ventures. But then Herschel Walker was always more than just one of the best running backs in the NFL. He has danced with the Fort Walker Ballet, served as the brakeman in a two-man bobsled at the 1992 Olympics, and earned a fifth-degree black belt in tae kwon do. And there is always that tennis match.

"I never read that you're only supposed to play football," says Walker. "That was just me, living."

Other athletes, like 1993 Cy Young Award winner Jack McDowell, gravitate to the creative arts. After retiring in 1999, McDowell formed a pop-alternative band called Stickfigure.

"I was pigeonholed as this certain type of person in baseball," McDowell told *Sports Illustrated.* "The person inside of me—the real Jack—was the person coming out in the songs."

Kym Hampton retired from the WNBA's New York Liberty in 1999 with a serious knee injury but landed a gig as a back-up vocalist on Luscious Jackson's album *Electric Honey*. Asked about her back-up role she told a reporter, "You have to start out right because you don't get a second chance." But isn't Hampton *making* a second chance in a pursuit that won't require world-class knees?

And what of Yannick Noah, the flamboyant French tennis player who won the 1983 French Open? These days you can find Noah as a front man for his reggae band Zam Zam, a tight group that has produced five albums over eleven years.

"Music is like therapy," He told *Sports Illustrated*. "The more I sing the better I feel."

That seems like a good compass: If it makes you feel better and is not detrimental to your health, follow it. Cross that bridge and don't look back.

Bjorn Borg is one who got stuck on the bridge. Borg shocked the tennis world in 1982 by announcing his retirement at the age of twenty-seven. He was at the top of his game, in superb physical condition, but unable to summon the motivation and willpower to stay on top of the Grand Slam circuit. It was January 15, 1981, at the Volvo Masters in New York City, and Borg was playing his nemesis and future friend John McEnroe. For the first time anyone could remember, Borg argued with the umpire and had a point deducted. Somehow the icy cold Swede appeared to have developed a crack in the veneer; he was human after all.

That summer he lost to McEnroe in the Wimbledon final and at the U.S. Open later that year. "I was so disappointed," he was quoted saying. "I thought it was the end of my life."

Borg was right: It was the end of his life, the beginning of the end of his professional tennis life. He had stepped onto that bridge.

While it would be nearly two years until he made his retirement official, Borg never found what had eluded him—the fiery will to succeed.

After a series of failed marriages, child custody suits, and business deals turned bad, Borg attempted to get off the bridge, to step back to the world of pro tennis where he had felt so secure and had been so successful.

As we've seen, though, a return to sport has to be for the pure love of it. If you go back for fame or money, your chances of finding happiness again in playing are slim.

Borg's return to tennis was doomed from the beginning. People laughed when he attempted to use his beloved wooden rackets against the aerospace-inspired unobtanium graphite composite weapons the other players were using. He lost to players who had been in diapers when he won the first of his eleven Grand Slam titles, players he would have dispatched in straight sets.

Eventually, though, Borg moved across the bridge while finding a new place in tennis: success on the senior circuit, a more light-hearted approach, a gradual acceptance of what he had meant to the game, and what the game had (and had not) meant to him.

When he finally left the senior circuit in 2001 it was with a sense of understanding and personal maturity that seemed lacking at the time of his first retirement nearly twenty years earlier.

"It wasn't until I stopped playing tennis," he quipped, "that I realized that in real life problems exist."

With this single admission, Bjorn Borg was discovering the way across. He was going where he needed to be.

A Day in the Life...or Lives

"I get up, I walk, I fall down. But through it all I keep dancing."

—Rabbi Hillel

The sixteen-year-old kid pounded on my front door. It was an authoritarian knock, more announcement than inquiry. I was upstairs changing my daughter's diapers. I looked out the window to see who the kid and his pimply-faced buddy in the beat-up Chevy Camaro were.

Geez, it's Lance, I thought. Shouldn't he be in school? Oh well, it's early June, maybe they let them out early in Texas. But how the hell did they get that car out here, and what's he doing at my house?

"Came out to train with the big boys," he said. "Gonna own this sport in a few years."

"That's great Lance. Come on in and see the four-month-old we own now. And tell your buddy to get that heap off my driveway before it leaks oil on the free-throw line."

My daughter, cleaned up and ready to rock, made a short *a* sound and looked at the kid with the deep brown eyes and short hair. Nobody in my family had short or brown hair. I of course told my visitor that she was trying to say "dad." To this day, Lance swears that my sixteen-year-old daughter's first word was "Lance."

Armstrong's story is well documented. There is little I can add other than to say that his brash and booming confidence, peppered with intelligence and loyalty, is the reason he is alive today. The greatest American cyclist in history (with a nod to Greg LeMond) will have no trouble when he leaves the sport. He has experienced death already.

He knows how to reinvent himself. He has every tool you could want when it comes to major life transition. No, Lance Armstrong, the cocky sixteen-year-old triathlete who left Plano High School and moved to San Diego to train with the best athletes in the sport, will not suffer when he puts the bike up in the rafters. He's had the practice. He has seen dark days and knows that the nature of bright sunlight is to cast long shadows. And he knows the circularity of life, that the sun also rises, that pain and suffering eventually become just an idea whose day has passed.

Fast forward fifteen years.

7:32 *A.M. Drive my sixteen-year-old daughter Torrie to school. The parking lot is full of BMWs and new VW Bug Cabriolets purchased by parents more divorced than married. I can sense the rising stress in Torrie as we near the pretentious school.*

"It's tough, isn't it Tor, thinking you have to keep up with all this stuff."

"Dad, you have no idea."

"What about a sport? I know you've tried lots of them but isn't there something that sounds as if you would like it, that would give you a feeling of accomplishment and self-esteem?"

"Dad, you've been trying to make me an athlete since you put me in pee-wee soccer at three years old. Face it, I'm not a jock. So just get over it!"

7:45 *A.M. Return home just in time to see my eleven-year-old son Dane walking off to school with a neighbor kid. His pants are pulled low and boxer shorts peak out like a symbol of rebellion.*

"Hey dude, how about a hug for the old man?"

"Ah Dad, I'm already late."

I stand in a vigil to the passing of the torch, looking at myself in a thirty-year-old mirror, our difference in ages, fighting to let go.

"Okay kiddo, see you after school. Luv ya."

But walking up to the front door I turn around to see Dane returning to hug his old man. And all is right with the world.

7:53 A.M. *Second cup of coffee. That's enough. Park myself at command central and turn on the box. Thirty-eight e-mails. No I don't want Viagra, a penis enlargement, a lower monthly mortgage payment, or a free trip to Las Vegas. Technology has not made my life easier. Even Tim Flannery has resorted to spam e-mails touting his next gig with so and so, the best percussionist in the county. I turn off the noise and return to a chapter of a novel I'm working on. It's about a Vietnam vet who is traveling the country trying to find the soul that the war took from him.*

8:01 A.M. *A friend calls and says Greg Welch is back in the hospital. His implanted defibrillator shocked him out of ventricular tachycardia six times yesterday. I hang up the phone and wonder where all the rules went. Imagine if you trained hard, ate right, and took care of yourself, if you did the right thing and treated people with kindness and respect, if you acted like, well, like Welchy. And now you're lying in a hospital bed, desperately trying to find hope and put on the positive face. But it's beat you down and beat you down, and order has turned into chaos, physical beauty and prowess into bodily anarchy. You're fucked up, and it pisses you off. It's not so much the illness that has you tweaked but the overwhelming ambiguity of it all. What would you do? What would I do? Welchy had already gone through a dozen major medical procedures and for all means and purposes, he was back at square one.*

I hang up the phone, make plans to go see him, and wonder why and how triathlon had screwed up our bodies. We were supposed to be the wonder-kids, the Ironmen who could do it all. "Look at them go," they'd all say, "Energizer bunnies. Nothing can stop those kids."

11:45 A.M. *The mail arrives and there is an invitation from the Ironman organizers inviting me to return this October for "the spectacular twenty-fifth anniversary" of the first running of the now-fabled event in Hawaii. It had been four years since I last raced there. They are offering to waive my entry fee and qualifications and to pay* *a travel stipend. I do some quick math and figure it will only cost me a grand or so to go over. I'm not in any shape to race and have no desire to watch, but I have these pangs of prodigal-son desire to see what would happen. I put the letter in a big pile and wait for something to happen. Maybe an idealized collection of the event's virtues will meld with my own selective memory and I can return to something fixed and permanent. But I already know too well the mind's fluidity, and so I return to my traveling vet novel. At least he could slip his old skin, like a molting snake shedding his nightmares, and just lie in the sun, warming his cold blood and growing a new future. Fiction is beautiful in that way. Then again, fiction always has a basis in reality, and this character has roots in me.*

1:13 P.M. I pack up my backpack and head up to campus. I have to hand in grades for my class, return books to the library, and thank a few profs for their help this term. It's been a tough but pivotal semester and I feel good about the work I did. I am lucky and I know it. There is something vibrant and visceral about college campuses. They remind me of sports stadiums in some ways— they are places of passion and movement and action and climax. And it happens over and over and over again. There are sexual undertones in both places.

4:45 P.M. Stuck in traffic on the way home. I'm reminded of the time when my car broke down while I was driving from San Diego to San Francisco and I put on a pair of running shoes and simply ran the ten miles to the nearest gas station. When traffic came to a complete halt I thought about pulling over, putting my running shoes on, and jogging home. The first person I would call would be Tom Warren. He would appreciate that. People are always saying to invest in this stock or that bond. What's so wrong about investing in yourself? If Alcatraz were still an active prison and I were sent there for leaving my car on the side of the road too many times, I would tell the guards, whatever you do, don't make me swim that mile and a half across those treacherous waters. I might drown.

5:35 P.M. *I go for a run and decide to take my dog Molly. She is almost fifty in dog years but runs like she's eighteen in human numbers. As I plod along the center of the trail, she zigzags with great speed and intent from bush to bush, flushing out rabbits, flushing out her day spent pacing the backyard as if she knew that at any moment she could die and wake up in the photo album of a family that liked to do what she did. Just not as much. I watch her frenetic but purposeful strides and wonder at the innocence and pleasure that pervades her motion. She doesn't know or care about the costs. She is alive and that is all that matters.*

6:36 P.M. *Virginia comes home from work while Dane and I are out on the trampoline. It's a dangerous toy but I am not innocent to that fact. We are having fun and that is all that matters. Dane calls for mom to come and join the fun. But groceries and dinner preparations and life get in the way. I don't offer to help. I'm a schmuck and I know it.*

7:28 P.M. *There's dinner dishes, kids' homework, a friend in the hospital to go see tonight, and in chapter nine my vet has just met an eight-year-old girl who will help heal some of his wounds. I wonder if I should sneak into the pool at the apartment complex down the street for a quick thousand yards but decide that would be just like the old me. Everything has changed and nothing has changed.*

11:17 P.M. *The house is quiet except for the sound of a south wind moving through the palm tree outside my office window. I'm rereading an English translation of Jacques Derrida's* Writing and Difference. *It is a dense and difficult combination of Western philosophy and oblique literary theory. I understand every other sentence, which is better than a year ago when only every third got through. I am training my mind as I did my legs and lungs. But I don't have the luxury of youth so I have fast-tracked myself. After Derrida, Foucault and Husserl will seem easy.*

11:46 P.M. *I try to fall asleep but am curious about the surreal and spiritual texture of the day. It was as if there had been a falling-away of the definite, as if something had happened and I had failed to notice, or perhaps I was afraid that something was going to happen and would pass me by. I did not expect good dreams.*

Letting Go

"As I get older, I'm finding that some things I felt were important are not. And others, like friendships that I've had and the people whose lives have touched mine, are omnipotent. You take for granted that they're going to be around for a long, long time, and that's not necessarily the case."
                                        —Notes from the author's diary

I cherished the first real bicycle I owned, a pearl-white ten-speed of some long-forgotten make. Six months, maybe a year, I worked odd and arduous jobs to save for that sleek machine. The $98 I spent on it seemed like a fortune considering our modest family budget. I kept it clean, well tuned, and locked in my bedroom until the day I was hit by a car as I ran a stop sign racing home for dinner. And at fourteen years old, carrying that jumble of scrap metal, rubber, and wire cable home like a soldier pulled from the battlefield, I had to stop and wipe the tears from my eyes before I walked in the door.

I was okay though, save for a grapefruit-sized bruise on my leg and a deep sense of remorse. The bike was a total loss. Dinner wasn't even ready.

Nearly a quarter century later, I came home from another short ride just in time for dinner and noticed four large cardboard boxes sitting on my front porch. Oh great, I yawned, my new bikes for the season are here. The custom machines were worth at least four grand a piece and I purposely let them sit there for three days before I dragged them into the garage one at a time and, over the course of a few weeks, pulled them out of their cradles. I wanted to see if the material aspect of sport still held any purchase with me. Slowly letting go of my sports equipment was part of my letting go of the sport. They were beautiful machines, but the realization that I may never really put them to their highest and best use was but one more test in seeing how far I'd come in moving past that life.

Real letting go comes at the end. It comes when that grip we have on sport, that grip it has on us, is finally pried away the only way it can be—one finger at a time.

It's a hard concept for some people to grasp, this connection to what they may perceive as a simple game. But it's there, undeniable, powerful enough to take some of the strongest, fittest, most courageous athletes of their time and lay them flat. Not like a linebacker's hit or a fifty-mile run. More like a persistent bill collector who won't leave you alone. Making it to the top ranks of a sport is not the hardest thing you will ever do. Stepping down and letting go is.

When you let go of the things that bind you to a career, a lifestyle, an identity, you do so in small and subtle ways. Sometimes you notice, other times you don't. There is never a sudden psychological and spiritual breaking of the ties. That is what healing from loss is all about; it is an acceptance that you will no longer have what you had, or be who you were. And you can only heal as fast as your body, your head, and your heart will let you. They are on a clock of their own.

If you have invested enough of yourself in the identity of the professional athlete, as most have, you never leave it completely. It may sound odd, but you are a survivor of sport. You are somebody who used to be somebody else, stronger, richer, more famous, faster, thinner, better-looking. You were immortal back then. Now you have to face the inevitable and ultimate loss—that of your old identity and the false protection it gave you from facing your own mortality. Maybe that's why we let go in small steps.

My acceptance of this loss came in fleeting moments, some painful, some liberating. At first I would fight them, confusing acceptance with weakness. When my competitive results started to slip, I trained harder, worked smarter, and relished the days I could beat guys half my age. But I would not accept the fact that I was any less of an athlete than I was six months ago, or on the good days, six years ago.

One of the more interesting things about the stages of loss is that they don't always come in order. Anger is often the first thing people feel: anger at the death of a loved one (Why him? He was so young), anger over a lost wallet (Stupid me! Where'd I leave it?), anger over a career-ending injury, anger over a missing restaurant order. Big losses, little losses, the initial reaction is often the same.

The classic stages as detailed by the work of Elizabeth Kubler-Ross are anger, denial, depression, bargaining, and acceptance.

Somehow I never got angry in the beginning of my exit. Perhaps my anger slowly dissipitated into guilt and remorse and even melancholy as the years of healing wore on. I used to wish that I could just throw one huge temper tantrum, bust up a few hotel rooms, maybe even get myself thrown in jail for a few nights. Then I would accept my loss and be okay once again. I guess I didn't have enough anger in me, or I had seen enough of it thrown at innocent bystanders that I chose to point what I had inward.

And then, even before the depression set in, before I began the bargaining stage, which in some ways an athlete never leaves, I began to experience moments of acceptance. I would look at all this beautiful, expensive triathlon equipment in my garage (my bikes were worth twice as much as my car) and it meant nothing to me.

I would think, "Great, I have my priorities right." But later, I would feel sad that I would never be able to race those bikes or shoes or wetsuits as fast as they had the potential to go.

But then one morning I would wake up early, pull one of those fancy titanium bikes off the rack, roll down the driveway wearing a pair of surf trunks and an old ratty T-shirt thinking that I earned this bike, and it runs just as smooth and quiet at eighteen miles per hour as it does at twenty-eight, and if I stopped at the store for a soda, came out, and found it gone, well, it had been a good ride all the same. Then I would save my money until I had the 2003 equivalent of $98 and go buy a bike to use more casually.

Emmitt Smith, the running back from the Dallas Cowboys, once spoke about the need for passion to play hard when it really counts.

"You need that passion to work out in the off-season," he said, "when you'd rather be playing with your kids."

I struggled with that for a long time. I knew I could always work out in the off-season, and that my kids would be grown and gone before I knew it. But I also knew that my off-seasons were even more limited than my years of raising children. I had to accept that many of the good things in life come in limited supply. Strong muscles, white teeth, innocence—they don't last forever. Then again, love, tolerance, and passion are ageless.

Yeah, acceptance is the hardest, so it takes the most time, it puts up the greatest fight, and if you allow it, it brings the greatest rewards. It's sort of a learned trait. You can talk about it, study it, get counseled in it, meditate, learn yoga, and drink only ginkgo biloba tea. In the end, the best you can do is recognize when it's happening in you. And then be very compassionate and gracious in the process.

When my wife and I were in college, the concept of the soup and salad bar was born. This modern capitalist version of the soup line was perfect for us. We could go and spend $2.49 each, one ordering soup and the other salad, switch plates mid-gorge, and eat a huge, healthy meal for five bucks and change. I would grab a handful of muffins, take one bite of each, and then roll them up in napkins to be stuffed in Virginia's purse. She would insist I was stealing food; I'd say that since they were going to throw them out anyway we might as well take them home and have them for breakfast. Of course, the crumbs would get all over her purse but I would heat the muffins up in the morning, put some butter on them, and the episode would be forgotten.

But the pattern was set. For over twenty years, whenever we stopped at one of those now commodified, yuppified, and institution-alized soup and salad places, I would eat like a pig. It wasn't the money (although the prices had risen fivefold) or the fact that my kids would eat only two baby carrots, half a slice of whole wheat bread, and two chocolate chip cookies. It was something else. I was a professional athlete. I trained really hard and had to abstain from too many sensory pleasures in my quest to go fast. I *deserved* to eat a big meal. Even if I wasn't hungry I would surround my place at the table with so many different plates that it looked like a model of the solar system.

Not long ago I took my kids to one of those soup and salad places. They now remind me of upscale hospital cafeterias, just gluttonous food factories for the I'm-too-busy-to-cook-had-a-late-meeting-let's-just-go-to-Salads-R-Us-tonight crowd. But the kids love them because they can run around, serve themselves, chat with their buddies, and pretend they had a healthy meal. While my son and daughter were doing just that, I helped myself to a small salad and one bowl of soup. plus a glass of shitty cabernet for an extra four bucks.

We ate, cleared our table, and got up to leave. As I held my son's hand walking across the parking lot, he asked if I was sick.

"No Dane, why do you ask?"

"Well Dad, you didn't eat very much."

It was then that I recognized a sign of acceptance: I didn't need a three-thousand-calorie gorge when I would only burn two thousand all day.

No son, I ate small because I think I'm getting better.

It's not easy to let go, mostly because you worked so hard to get there. But athletes do, and some do it with dignity and grace.

You're supposed to get smarter as you get older. But how old is old? Tennis star Michael Chang is only thirty, but he has been playing professionally for almost fifteen years—half of his life. He speaks of fellow players Andre Agassi and Pete Sampras as "the older American boys."

"You know," said Chang, "we've been playing on tour for quite some time...they know that we're not going to be playing for five or ten more years. Obviously, all of us would like to be able to go out on a high note. I think that's any professional athlete's dream."

The dream rarely comes true. More often than not, athletes play out their last days in a state of quiet brooding submission. They play less and less, their confidence eroding with time.

Some of them, like Mark Messier, the forty-two-year-old captain of the New York Rangers, fight their decline as most people would fight their own early death. Even with the fans and the press calling for retirement, players like Messier will not go quietly into that good night. Acceptance for them is to work harder, work smarter, keep performing where you can, and ignore the calls to step down.

Indeed, many star players who have been training and eating properly in the off-season throughout their careers are knocking down the conventional age barriers. Barry Bonds hit seventy-three home runs at thirty-seven years old. At thirty-nine New York Yankees ace Roger Clemens went 20–1 and claimed a sixth Cy Young Award. In hockey, goalie Patrick Roy, age thirty-six, posted four shutouts in five games for the Colorado Avalanche, the defending Stanley Cup champions. Detroit defenseman Chris Chelios, thirty-nine, and forwards Steve Yzerman and Brett Hull, thirty-six and thirty-seven, respectively, led the Red Wings to one of the best records in the NHL in 2001.

Maybe these guys looked at wide receiver Jerry Rice, who caught eight touchdown passes at thirty-nine years old, or Nolan Ryan, who was still throwing ninety-five-mile-per-hour fastballs at forty-five, or Hockey Hall of Famer Gordie Howe, who played twenty-six seasons (plus six in the WHA) and endured 1,767 NHL games, scoring 801 goals and winning four Stanley Cups with the Red Wings. All before retiring at age fifty-two.

Maybe part of an athlete's acceptance is that if they *can* still play, and play well, they *must*. What motivates them becomes their own business. They still have that passion or they still love the game or maybe they need the money. It might be that by remaining in the game for as long as they can, they create a direct link from one generation of players to the next, in keeping with that folk refrain, "may the circle remain unbroken."

I once sat next to the legendary tennis star Roy Emerson at an awards banquet. I've talked about driving fast with Danny Sullivan, played basketball with the great NFL lineman Bob Golic, raced Roger Craig and Vinny Testaverde in a one-hundred-yard dash, watched Dick Fosbury (of the Fosbury Flop) cut his front lawn, took a leak next to Steve Garvey, skied with Billy Kidd, talked about raising kids with Cal Ripken, Jr., accepted a gift of bike pedals from five-time Tour de France winner Bernard Hinault, jumped off a boat to swim from Alcatraz to the sidewalks of San Francisco with Doug Flutie, rode my bike with Bill Walton, and told Lance Armstrong's mother that we would "watch over him" when he showed up at a triathlon at fifteen years old.

I don't say this to drop names but to remind myself that I have grown up with three generations of legendary sports figures. These chance meetings and friendships mark a kind of family tree in which I can place myself, maybe not as a famous competitor but as a small branch somehow connected to a large trunk of history. I suppose someday that connection will mean something to me. I will read an obituary and a tear will form in my eye because I bought a few beers for a sports hero and a friend, just a couple of beers. And now he is dead.

Letting go of your life's love is like letting go of your parents or your spouse; when you were younger, you just knew they would always be there. Kevin Lowe played hockey his whole life, including many years in the NHL, mostly for the Edmonton Oilers. He thinks he has let go, but Kevin Lowe is still a hockey player, maybe more than ever, as he guides other teams in a managerial position.

"People would ask 'What are you going to do next?' and I didn't even want to think about it," he said. "I'm just going to focus on the last two or three years of my playing. I'm not even going to worry about that. Next year is next year. I'm playing this year and I'm focused on that. You really try to not think too far ahead. It was easier for me—it's like signing a contract, you don't want to sign two years because one year gives you focus but it doesn't give you the security; it gives you the energy to play hard, because you try to play an extra year and do all the right things, but also subliminally it says, 'If I want, I can just walk away from this year,' and every time I went on the ice it was sort of like…'This could be my last game that I will ever play in the NHL.'"

Maybe some athletes hang on as long as they can because they can't think of another damn thing they'd rather be doing. So they accept the fact that they will play as long as some yardstick tells them they should. They know that obit will be there one day.

Or if they can't play, they can pretend. There is a great distance between athletes who hang on for the love of the game, or to give something back, and athletes who don't really compete anymore but have convinced themselves that somehow, in some way, they are still in it, still a part of the crew. The party was over hours ago but there are always a few guests who hang around; they don't have any place else to go, any place else where they feel at home. So they stay until the host reminds them that they don't really live there. It's sad but sometimes it's better to throw them out the door, force them to fish or cut bait, to get a life. And a new one at that.

Every sport has its late-night set, its hangers-on. They are easily identified by the sport-specific markers they continue to wear until they wear out. Baseball has its chewing tobacco, basketball its trash talk, skiing has fashion, and surfing its gnarly vernacular. In triathlon we had shaved legs.

You see the old retired dogs dressing the part, throwing out the radar for all the world to see and know that, yes, they too are still part of the tribe, if only in ritual—that's when pity steps in and says, well, maybe it's not a lie but there's enough white noise around to cover up any truth. If they've earned it, I say let them live out any fantasy that gives them comfort.

Borrowed from swimming, shaving your legs (or your whole body if the race is really big or your self-esteem is really low) supposedly enables you to move faster through the water. Cyclists will also shave their legs under the guise that if they crash, the chances of infection around the road-rash wound are less with smooth, hairless skin. So if you want the world to know you are a triathlete, shaved legs can be worn as a badge.

All this makes perfect sense and is backed by a certain amount of empirical truth in addition to the placebo effect. I shaved my legs for years, never truly buying the whole shtick but thinking that if I didn't, I would be giving something away to my competitors. It's part of the pre-race ritual, no different than war paint or kamikaze sake ceremonies. There are those who just aren't meant to let go easily. Some warriors die old and die well and are buried still with a spear in their hands.

From Body to Mind: The Redirection of Self

"Die so that you can live."

—Johann Wolfgang von Goethe

Each person has his or her own genius. For a housewife it might be taking care of her kids. For the businessperson it's about profit and success. For creative types, developing their unique gifts. And for athletes like the legendary pitcher Satchel Paige, it's about doing things with the body that are beyond the scope of everyday athleticism.

A friend's grandfather once batted against the great Paige. He told his grandson that he was just another man who could be considered the best pitcher of all time.

For top athletes, who at an early point in life seem to have fulfilled their individual genius, the problem is that once your gift is no longer your compass, the fire that fuels your days, you are just another person who might be considered the best there ever was. Ironically, that syndrome applies to all "geniuses." For the lifelong mother, an empty house can be terrifying. The twenty-eight-year-old dot.com millionaire may have achieved her goal but lost her dream.

"You need a reason to get up every day," NFL star Ronnie Lott told the writer Bill Lyon, "otherwise, you have this feeling of being empty. You have to find a purpose for living."

The operational word is "find." For the athlete, whose connection to the world was primarily through his or her body and its gifts, the first impulse is to find another way to use the body to define identity.

But that only works in a few cases, and often for a short period. Where then does one find purpose for living?

The next stop must be upstairs, in the head. That is where I ended up, not on purpose but because it was necessary for my happiness, my future, and dare I say it, my survival as a sane, well-adjusted individual.

Having been a writer for some time, or at least a guy who put words on a page to try and make sense of his thoughts, I began to write, a lot. First it was just notes on a page, ideas, thoughts, confessions, and notes from my few talks with a "retirement counselor," just some hidden way of saying I sought professional help. Then I would string together short essays for other athletes who wrote to me for advice. Finally I began to create fictional stories, stories filled with tragedy and loss, realism and pathos just dripping off the page.

What interested me was the way I felt when I wrote: It was as if my fractured sense of self would temporarily come together in the momentary act of creation. The anxiety that had stemmed from my lack of direction subsided in those precious moments when I projected thoughts and ideas as characters in a plot. When I wrote, I was well. I could say anything, be anybody, explore, travel, cry, hate, make love, heal or be healed, kill or be killed, rebel or accept. I could be absolutely honest with myself.

And as I did, the truth began to emerge and my ability to feel returned. I realized in a kind of catharsis that I had lost the ability to feel the way I had before my life in sport. Somehow all the focus on *me*, on what was necessary for *my* career, had robbed me of that which makes us human—feelings of compassion and pain and unadulterated joy and a thousand other emotions. Maybe it was a protective device that crept in after all those years of grueling, day-long training sessions. Maybe my narcissism had just run amuck as it does in so many professional athletes. And quite possibly there was a physiological element to my feeling-less state.

If all our thoughts and feelings have a corresponding chemical state in the brain, it makes sense to suppose that a person whose body chemistry has been compromised by illness, injury, or long-term stress might not have a normal capacity to feel emotion. An athlete who had subjected himself to years of arduous training might fall into this category.

I discussed this with my friend Dr. P. Z. Pearce, and he not only agreed but claimed that the theory had been his idea and I had somehow appropriated it through all our conversations. He is probably correct and if he gets a Nobel Prize for science, I begrudge him nothing.

"But P. Z.," I would barb him, "all you scientist guys come up with ideas and theories and such. I'm the guy who's living through this, who's, feeling it, or should I say, not feeling it."

"S. T.," he would reply, "you're just as much a scientist as I am, all this reading and research and interviewing you're doing. That's not exactly an outdoor play activity." He was right, about the play, not about my being a scientist type. I was just looking for answers.

In any case, we played with various medications that affected the levels of neurotransmitters (those chemicals that help us feel things) and the results were somewhat inconclusive. I still believe that endurance athletes who submit themselves to chronic overtraining are susceptible to altered, mostly depressed, states of emotion. Someday if we can come up with a practical way to measure serotonin (which can be measured through a spinal tap), dopamine, and epinephrine, the three primary identified agents, we may be able to gauge the psychological effects of overtraining.

These were the kinds of things I thought about and dreamt about. As I lay in bed late at night making those soft pig noises of sleep, my wife would wake me up and claim that I had been calling out names of other athletes in my dreams. "Who were they?" I'd ask.

"I don't know. But all the guys' names ended in 'zine.'"

Ah shit, I thought, I'd been dreaming about some new wonder drug that would answer all my problems. Just when I thought I was getting through denying my problems were physiological, I was confusing medication with meditation.

So I would go to the place where I could dream during the regular hours of day, the only place where no one could get to me by phone or e-mail or screaming up the stairs or carrier pigeon or mental telepathy.

I would paddle out into the ocean until I could see the edge of the coast bend and turn.

There I would sit, two, three, five miles out on my twelve-foot paddle board, and listen to the current moving in sync with the wind and the clouds, the waves lapping up against the side of my board, watching the answers flow in as the moon and the sun watch the tide.

Sport had offered much, but there was so much more to life. I had betrayed myself into thinking I had balance in my life. I had betrayed others in thinking that I needed to train eight hours a day when some of that was pure fun. My sport was narcissistic. I had been passionate about it, but partially because my passion had no other outlets—outlets that I needed to find now.

I suddenly realized that as Westerners, we are defined by what we do, not by who we are. If I could go to Nepal for a few years and train with Buddhist monks, I might be able to fully accept the fact that we are who we are, no matter what we do and how we surround ourselves with people, responsibilities, or material possessions.

An airline pilot is forced to retire after flying for thirty-three years, and he complains to his psychiatrist that he feels lost, without meaning or purpose. He would do well to consider that he will always be who he is, regardless of how he spends his days. There is only one of him. When he flew that plane, he had people's lives in his hands. He was needed, he was important. When he wakes up on a cold January day and has nowhere to go, nothing to do but take out the trash and balance the checkbook, it is no wonder he feels lost. His plane has left without him because, in the company's eyes, he is too old to be effective and safe.

The pilot first needs to let the plane go and realize he will never again command a 747. He may choose to rent a Cessna 172 and buzz around the county with a few friends, no different than Cal Ripken, Jr. throwing the ball with the neighborhood kids. But the sooner he can let it go and find something else to lift his spirits, the sooner he will find a way to replace that plane.

On that day, I paddled in and went looking for my old friends.

▼ ▼ ▼

For athletes to truly recognize what sport has meant to them, they must become aware of their personal horizons. And ultimately they must realize that those planes of existence will be temporary if they are simply self-centered.

How shallow is an unshared victory? Dave Debusschere, forward for the New York Knicks, once told a reporter that, "When you're through playing, when you're older, you go back to your friends." That's where you go...and you give back.

There are hundreds of examples of professional athletes giving selflessly of their time, effort, and money, both while they are playing and when they retire. Their motives are as varied as the causes they support. But they all have realized that they are part of the human race, not just a running or cycling race.

Former heavyweight boxing champion Ken Norton was so moved by one visit to a home for abused children that he started a foundation called World Champions Against Abuse.

Most people will agree that any famous person who is highly paid for his or her fame, regardless of how it was earned, has a responsibility to help those who are less fortunate. I think that the athletes' responsibility to help others is also a responsibility to themselves. There is so much healing in the healing of others.

"How come you don't tell the class about when you were a professional athlete? I mean, like, I would be so proud if I had won all those races."

I was packing up my books and lecture notes from the table in front of the classroom. This valid question was coming from a nineteen-year-old woman who was in the Intro to Creative Writing class I was teaching at San Diego State University.

The young writer had been in one of my previous classes and we had become friends; she knew more about my past than most of my professors and fellow grad students. At some point I had tried to make it clear that my new life as a writer and a teacher and student of sociology and psychology of sport was separate from what came before. And I needed that separation.

But I hadn't elaborated, thinking there was no reason to. She's nineteen. What does anyone know about leaving a past behind at nineteen? Still, it was an interesting question, one that I thought I could answer. Or maybe not.

"Just tell the class you were a jock then and a teacher guy now. They'll think it's pretty cool."

Yes, they might think it was "pretty cool" and then they might wonder how I could know the craft of creative writing, the intricacies of fiction, the elemental power and potential of poetry. How could I teach them to develop voice and tone and style, to work with flashback and foreshadow, if for the last twenty years I had been focused on the improvement of the body? I couldn't take the chance. I'd let my students figure out my past if they wanted (some of them did and brought it up), and if the subject never came up, well, there was plenty to cover in the fifteen weeks of the semester. I loved teaching.

Fiction was a place where I could explore my past and dabble in my future, a place where I could be somebody I wasn't, test-drive new ideas, and discard old baggage. When I wrote fiction, all these things came together in the single moment called *now*. It was, and always is, the special place that the psychoanalyst D. W. Winnicott called the "transitional phenomenon." Sport had kept me always looking around the corner. My time in transition had forced me to look back for awhile. The present is where it's all happening.

The best thing I could do in my efforts to reintegrate myself was to share with a few eager young minds the techniques and lessons I had learned in my years of writing. I wondered if there were other athletes who had played at a world-class level and then ventured into a highly cerebral environment. I knew it was hard, simply from my own experience. You don't piggyback on what you've learned in sport. You have little or no credibility in the classroom; your background in sport can have an adverse effect.

Gradually I found a few. There was Michael Oriard, the English professor who had played in the NFL with the Kansas City Chiefs, and my old rowing coach Steve Estes. Lidia Yuknavitch, an early writing professor of mine, is a charismatic women and top-shelf writer who was a member of the 1980 Olympic swimming team. I never knew she had been a world-class swimmer until it slipped out one day. There was Doug Barba, who just missed a chance to pitch in the majors when he threw his arm out; instead he returned to school for a doctorate and a position teaching sport psychology at a West Coast university. There was Tom Meschery, the former NBA player who played alongside Wilt Chamberlain the night Wilt scored one hundred points. Today Tom is a published poet who teaches high school English and who is also married to the novelist Joanne Meschery. He is one of the few who has experienced success both in the ultimate physical world of pro sports and in the arts. And there was my friend Jerry Sherk, formerly of the Cleveland Browns, who went on to receive a master's in psychology.

I was telling Jerry the story of the young student who had prodded me to tell the class about my past. We were sitting in an old minivan parked under a large pepper tree in the parking lot behind a pancake house.

"This is where I sometimes come to think," Jerry told me. "You know, when it gets a little busy around the house and I need to get out."

I thought of the term "disposable hero." Sherk had been one of the best in the league, an All Pro team member. Now he was running a business called Mentor Management, mostly helping troubled youth find their way in life. On occasion you could tell that Jerry still wrestled with his own place in life. He had done what he was supposed to do—play football. Now he was doing what he had to do. This part was more important to him, though maybe not to his fans. That's why we were sitting in the parking lot of a small shopping center, talking about our former lives in a beater with a missing hubcap. There was no corner office with a view or a TV studio with three cameras rolling, just two tired old warriors trying to figure it all out.

"So Jerry, you must know what I'm talking about. You've taken a much more mature perspective to looking at this whole thing. With the knowledge you've gained, how would you have approached your exit from sport and your adjustment in transition differently than what you did?"

"I don't know if I have a real good answer for that. Maybe, it could be an athlete's training that tells him the past is the past. I always try to stay even now. Good things happen out of competition as they do in competition. An extreme example of that is the baseball player who hits a home run and doesn't get too high. Then he is struck out ten times in a row, and doesn't get too low.

"I don't know what I would have done differently. I almost think, now that you bring it up, that I did the same thing in my post-career life that I did during my career—I didn't allow myself safety nets. I thought that without trying to act like I'm super-intelligent, because I don't think I really planned it—it wasn't a conscious decision. I put myself in some rough spots where I have to work through stuff, and now I have to work for a living. But I've learned enough to help others in my business mentoring people."

"Jerry, isn't that the concept of the 'wounded healer' that Joseph Campbell talks about? Where, according to mythology, the hero is wounded, maybe in a battle, and is sent away from the tribe to heal himself and then either returns healed, with the knowledge of how to heal others, or he dies alone in the forest by himself?"

"Exactly. I think that's kind of what life is about for me. It's about being wounded and learning how to work through things, and like you talked about, the journey is then somehow bringing part of that to somebody else. So I think in part that's what I'm doing."

"Maybe that was why the girl, who is quite spiritual, wanted me to share my past with the other students."

"Scott, the whole athletic experience rocks you at such a deep level, it rocks you on a level right to your belief in God. And it used to be that when things were going right, I thought, 'Well, I have this really cool relationship with God,' you know? And I promised Him that I would do certain things and in return he's given me this wonderful life. And then, with this integration of your bodily and mental skills in such a short period of time, you realize that whatever agreement you had with Him, if you did have an agreement, it isn't the one that you thought!"

"It seems that many of the answers we seek, Jerry, have to do with trying to combine Western and Eastern philosophy. As Westerners, we are so definition- and occupation-based. You know, you are what you work at. But there are people who ask the deeper questions, and these are deep questions—I mean the existentialist gig about our nature of being, it changes your typical Western Judeo-Christian dogma, like, okay, there's life after death, and if you're good you go to heaven."

"Yeah, and you have to go to church and there's an ecumenical foundation that you have to follow through and a new type of theory and belief system. Whereas the Eastern thought is that you are who you are at any one given moment. It doesn't matter what you're dealing with, you still have a soul and a foundation. But on the other side there's this kind of disintegration, this polarity of life that has as much to do with goodness as anything else."

"For sure. And if it circles back to mythology, it's got to be about death and dying. That's the thing in us that balances our struggle to exist and live to the fullest. You could also relate it to our subconscious desire to make war. And since war is pretty unpopular right now, to the embrace of violent sports. Did you ever feel that need Jerry, you know, to go to battle?"

"Oh yeah. You have that motivation to win but at the same time, you want that nurturing while you're a player, but just a little bit, you know? When you get injured, you get knocked down, you don't have a good game, you feel alienated from the rest of your friends and fans and society. And that whole syndrome gets amplified when you retire. You act a certain way and someone asks, 'What are you—a twelve-year-old?' Well, in some ways you *are* a twelve-year-old."

Suddenly, I had this image of when I was so depressed I could barely get out of bed in the morning. The only relief I found was in sleeping or putting myself at risk in the exposure to dangerous natural elements, long paddles into the ocean, surfing big waves alone, taking off and wandering around at night in a storm. I remember feeling like I needed to get out of bed in the morning and go back to being the Great Provider. But all I really wanted was for someone to come into my room, lie down next to me, and tell me it was going to be okay.

And it never happened. Besides a few phone calls from close friends, some hugs from my kids who didn't know why their dad didn't feel like playing, and small efforts to understand by my wife, I had to pull myself out of the dark alone. It was, and will always remain, the single greatest accomplishment in life.

I was going to tell part of the story to Jerry, but he beat me to it.

"Sometimes I think about when I moved back here from Cleveland and I have this kind of imagery of the experience going from this big strong hero to...I don't know, someone small. I can remember when I was married to the wife that I had when I was playing ball, and she started having other interests. And I was like this pathetic little character, and she'd come home and I'd been going through all these thought processes of how I'd hang on to her, and she's really great and I'm just a little pile of nothing. And I can literally remember saying stuff like, 'Well, I thought about it today, and while you're off doing this other thing, I'm just going to make it nice for you around here.' How pathetic? You know, like, 'Around these steps I'm gonna plant a shrub over here,' and 'When you come home I'll have some dinner waiting on the stove.' And I just thought, how pathetic is that, to be this hero and then almost immediately you're just this blubbering pile of jelly? I didn't realize that I needed to see myself as that wounded athlete. And to heal myself first."

But Jerry Sherk did, and he does more now in a month to better humanity than he did in a dozen seasons tackling quarterbacks in front of ninety thousand people. He is no longer a professional athlete, but he will always be a former player who used his body to its greatest potential. And who now uses his heart and mind in an even greater role.

Makings of a Transition

*"I feel great. I haven't had a bad day. I love life. I love living.
I work out every morning. By 7:30 I'm up banging the
weights and running."*
—Magic Johnson, 2002

hy do some athletes dance gracefully from a lengthy career in professional sports to a career in something different? How is it that someone like two-sport All Star Bo Jackson can be forced out of professional sport after only playing for ten years, the last three as a shadow of his former greatness after hip replacement surgery in 1991, and then find contentment with his business interests and family? And how is it that Mike Webster, the NFL Hall of Fame center for the Pittsburgh Steelers when they were the most dominant team in the league, a guy who played a full and rewarding career, ended up having trouble dealing with every problem life could throw at him? Webster, arguably the best center in the history of the NFL and by all accounts a simple, hard-working guy, was debauched of his wealth by former business partners, was separated from his wife, suffered undiagnosed health problems, and slept in his car when he couldn't afford a hotel room. How does this happen? How is it that Denver quarterback John Elway enjoyed what most reporters described as a "storybook retirement" and then went on to one of the most difficult periods of his life less than two years later?

And what makes a guy like Jim Tyrer, the All-Pro offensive tackle for the Kansas City Chiefs, shoot his wife and himself to death with a thirty-eight-caliber handgun when everyone thought Jim was "such a stable and together guy"?

Of course there is no one answer; each situation is unique and fluid. But there are patterns that can give clues on how an athlete might deal with his or her exit from sport.

Most athletes carry certain personality traits that enable them to achieve what they do in sport: work ethic, perseverance, focus, creativity, dedication. Those are the good things that will help in retirement. But athletes can also be obsessive, controlling, angry, self-centered, and manipulative. While these traits may help win football or hockey games, they will come back to haunt you when you leave sport. That which makes you great, can kill you in the end.

Many professional athletes may not even know their true selves all that well. If they started playing very early, as most do these days, then they grew up in an insulated world. They haven't been tested in ways that others have. How would they handle a sick and screaming child? Having to cut out coupons to buy enough food for the family? Getting laid off of a job? Professional athletes can do things we can only dream of. But the regular person can do things that athletes may struggle with.

They say that baseball players have it the worst. Most baseball players spend six or eight months a year playing ball and little else. And they have been doing it since the second grade. What could be so bad about this? It was their choice, and the ones who make the show will be taken care of in just about every way you can imagine. Millions of kids dream about playing major league baseball. What they don't dream about is having to retire from playing baseball. With all that "support" and assistance, how is a player supposed to learn how to do things like balance a checkbook, fix a leaky faucet, or discipline a teenage daughter? The truth is that most ball players do just fine. But for an athlete in a sport like field hockey, where a discount at the local sporting goods store constitutes a nice "salary package," the return to the real world of car problems and noisy neighbors will be easier.

The smarter athletes use the tools they developed playing sports to move into a new life. Magic Johnson played with a kind of charisma that no other player has matched, even Michael Jordan. That same charisma no doubt has served him well in the development of a growing business empire. NFL defensive star Ronnie Lott has an incredible ability to focus on the task, to get the job done. This focus led to 1,161 tackles in a fourteen-year career. When he retired, Lott had a hunch that he would be in trouble unless he kept moving.

"You try to exhaust things in life, do everything to the fullest," he told journalist Bill Lyon, "and then maybe you won't have time for regrets."

Today Lott works at half a dozen jobs, most of them for companies he owns or has founded. The others are charity gigs; giving back is part of the athlete's journey Lott has followed.

Rob Machado, one of the most popular professional surfers of all time, who is also a musician, a new father, and just about the mellowest guy you could ever meet, doesn't seem to question his fate in semi-retirement. He appreciates what he has, how hard he has had to work for it—and is all too happy to go along for the ride.

"I think surfing is different than any other sport, because right now, I just signed a new contract, and they don't care if I compete, you know?" No Rob, I don't know. But it sounds good to me. Where do we sign up? All they care about is for Rob to be himself and well, if it help sells product, well…all the better.

Team players generally have a harder time than single-sport athletes. The team becomes a family—perhaps more than a family, since few families go through what pro team players experience together. When you leave the team, the loss is profound, no different than losing a blood relative.

"You call the play, you break the huddle," remembers NFL Hall of Famer Steve Largent. "There's a sense of unity even in the clapping hands as you break the huddle together. In that respect, it is really a very, very unique experience in our society and culture today."

By contrast single-sport athletes, endurance athletes in particular, have usually spent an enormous amount of time alone in training. Retirement can bring them closer to their families or loved ones. But it can also toss them into a dark period because they simply don't have a network of close friends to both celebrate and mourn their career with.

Greg LeMond recalls when he first left the sport that had consumed so many years of his life.

"Well, I went through some depression, and I was kind of, you know, I just let myself go. Just saying, 'What the hell am I exercising for?' It wasn't the retirement I envisioned. I envisioned a retirement of one or two years of just doing everything I missed in my cycling career, the stuff that I loved to do but was never really able to do to its fullest. In reality I threw myself into stuff that just occupied my time and tried new things that might replace what I had in cycling, even as I became a new person."

I too had trained and raced in various forms: as a single guy, a married guy, a married father, and a married father with older kids—and each period had its own pluses and minuses. I missed my wife terribly at times; other times I was happy to have a few days on my own. Same with the kids. For several years, we dragged our daughter Torrie with us to events all over the world. She had filled up an entire passport before she was two years old. It seemed, and was at certain periods, a very nice arrangement.

But when Torrie asked me if we were ever going to live in a real house instead of a hotel, I knew it was time for her to start setting down roots.

The advantage that single-sport athletes have is that they can, if they choose, continue to practice their sport in some fashion. Greg LeMond can go out and ride his bike for twenty easy miles. He can ride for four or five hours if he is in shape and chooses to. Professional bike racing is very tactical and team oriented at the top levels, but the simple act of riding a bicycle is not.

Michael Jordan might be able to have a basketball game organized for him five days a week. But that's because he's Michael. Take a former NHL goalie. What's he going to do if he has a burning desire to feel again what it's like when the puck sinks deeply and contentedly into that big leather mitt? Will he go out and rent an ice rink and round up a handful of good players to take shots on him? Will he do this in the early evening between helping his son with homework and eating dinner?

How about a race car driver or a bobsled driver or a boxer? The greater the logistics of a sport, the harder it is to maintain your relationship with it. That's one reason why some pro players will not pick up a ball or bat for many years after their last real game. If they can't have it like it once was, why have it at all?

And some athletes, like the greatest Super Cross rider of all time, Jeremy McGrath, know they've missed the opportunity to go out on top—if indeed they share Michael Chang's opinion that this is "every pro's dream." So they settle for going out in one piece.

Motor sports like stadium Super Cross and motocross are riddled with ex-riders whose only wheels are now attached to a chair. Most of them, like David Bailey, are a constant presence on the off-road racing circuit. They are a reminder that *this* is what is waiting for you if fate or fear or a moment's indecision befalls you. A smart guy like McGrath knows this and avoids that thought for as long as he can. He knows that in a young and dangerous sport like Super Cross, when fear sets in it's time for you to step out. When he retired in the early spring of 2003 at thirty-one, it was with a record total of seventy-two Super Cross wins, money in the bank, a mostly healthy body, and no regrets.

"I'm happy with my decision," he told the *San Diego Union-Tribune*, "But in the back of my mind, I was always waiting for the sign that would tell me when to quit." McGrath received not one but two signs: a dislocated hip from a fall in practice and a new uneasiness about mixing it up with the leaders in several European Super Cross events.

It's hard to say how McGrath will handle retirement (he has a four-year contract with a motorcycle manufacturer to help build up its racing team). But the fact that he competed in a sport that, like bicycle racing, has both individual and team aspects may give him a unique perspective as he watches his career disappear in the rearview mirror.

On the other hand, having the opportunity to make a slow, gradual exit, as you can in individual sports, also means that you have the opportunity to view your own decline in slow motion. You can watch yourself miss jumps you used to make, get beat by kids you used to ignore, take minutes longer to get to the top of a hill. Players of highly physical sports also have a tough time, but for different reasons. Their bodies take a tremendous beating. Many NFL players retire with serious, chronic injuries that will never fully heal. It's one thing to retire and have to go through a few months or a year of "adjustment" problems, but to be reminded of your glory days every morning by a throbbing knee or a clicking ankle held together by enough titanium to set off an airport metal detector—well, that's enough to drive you back to the obsessive behavior you've been trying to control.

Football players once played in front of very large crowds of screaming, worshiping fans. Jerry Sherk put it this way: "When I played I was used to having that weekly dose of hearing ninety thousand fans. But when I retired, I asked my wife at the time to become those ninety thousand fans."

It's no wonder that the divorce rate for former NFL players is well over 50% within eighteen months of retiring. As former Chicago Bears player and coach Mike Ditka once said, "I couldn't exist without football." A lot of marriages can't exist without football either.

And what of that unique "war sport" called boxing? A contest that Jeffrey Sammons, in his influential book *Beyond the Ring*, argues is "directly associated with American strength and spirit," a sport that "has been effectively packaged, marketed, and sold as a natural activity possessing redeeming social values ranging from socioeconomic escalation to character building." What are we to make of the ubiquitous anecdotes of tragedy about retired boxers?

Boxers take a tremendous beating if they have successful careers; recent studies have confirmed long-term brain damage in career boxers. It doesn't mean they all will meet with tragic endings, but some do.

"A pioneering 1973 study," reports Sammons, "found that championship fighters often suffered the most brain damage because they met the toughest opponents, had longer careers, and consequently took more blows to the head." I have bouts of skin cancer on my face from training for so many years out in the sun. But the inside of my head seems to function fine.

Boxers pay a lot and don't often reap in-kind rewards. Unofficial records show that since 1884 approximately five hundred people have died in the ring worldwide. A 1980 study suggested that boxing is the deadliest contact sport. "Newspaper stories and word-of-mouth tales about the lucrative sums allegedly earned by boxing champions have often obscured reality," writes Sammons. Although the situation has improved in recent times, Sammons uses statistics from 1932 to show that New York boxing clubs paid out close to $1,500,000 to 945 boxers, giving them on average about $1,500 each, "a sum not far from the poverty line."

Boxing—how does one even begin to address the question of boxers retiring without spending chapters noting all the socio-cultural, psychological, and philosophical implications of two men (and now women) standing in a ring and beating the shit out of each other while thousands or millions of fans watch and bet money and cheer, wishing they could walk away with even a small percentage of a big fight's payday? Indeed, boxing offers one of the more direct parallels between sport and war; it is a reflection of the darker side of our society, yet also evidence of our society's ability to limit aggression to a small, controlled arena, a place they call the "squared circle."

Boxing, more than any sport, addresses the great decisions that a man must face at certain periods. The great Archie Moore, who fought a young Cassius Clay when he was forty-seven, said of the future Ali after one of the pre-fight debates, "I view this man with mixed emotions. Sometimes he sounds humorous but sometimes he sounds like Ezra Pound's poetry. He's like a man who can write beautifully but doesn't know how to punctuate. He has this twentieth-century exuberance but there's bitterness in him somewhere."

Moore, it was rumored, fought Clay at the time because he needed the money. And Muhammad Ali continues to fight, albeit a different type of opponent. Moore, for his part, fought his last bout at fifty years old in 1963 and retired with 141 career knockouts, more than any other boxer in history. He died in 1998 at nearly eighty-five, long-lived for a boxer. Both Ali and Moore exemplified the fight to close deep divisions that a man must deal with upon retirement, one by delaying that fight, the other by fighting an opponent he did not choose and which will chase him around life's "squared circle" until he is dead and the world mourns The Greatest.

The great boxer Sonny Liston's sparring partner Ray Schoeninger said this about Liston: "Many times I was around with Liston and he said, 'You like me, don't you?' Like a kid would." Liston's friend and corner man Davey Pearl said, "The thing with Sonny was that no matter how close you got to him—and we were close—you always got the feeling that there was sadness there that he wouldn't talk about."

I myself have been told that I write well but have poor spelling, literally and figuratively; that I seem content and fulfilled but there is an underlying sadness that is only perceptible when I am happy.

While they are playing, professional athletes need a little attachment for security and a lot of space to do their job. When they retire, that need gets reversed: They need people around them, people to take the place of the cheering crowd.

"People who need people," said sportswriter Dave Anderson, "don't retire." But not many people want to or could take the place of a cheering crowd. The best people to have around are others who have gone through something similar, something tragic, some event in which they too needed others to heal them.

When I retired, my wife was confused, often angry, and disappointed with me. I had been the alpha-male provider. Now I stayed up late, read or wrote constantly, and talked in a new language that intimidated her. It took me a long time to empathize with her. I was changing, I was not there—I was the problem. My friends were fellow grad students, professors, or kids from the beach. I was attracted to people who had suffered; I felt like a war vet in search of other vets. In fact, I began to study war and to write about it, fictional pieces about vets in search of themselves. I knew the protagonists well, but I could only move the narrative along as they began to heal through their experiences with others like them.

I'd run into an old friend whom I hadn't seen in many years and he'd ask, "Geez, so you're not racing triathlons anymore, eh? Must be great not to have to train so hard. What are you doing? Coaching? Television commentary? Doing the golf and public speaking circuit?"

No, I'd reply. I'm doing just what I did before I got into the sport twenty years ago: going to school, teaching and lifeguarding down on the beach. That was where I was finding my attachment: at school with other grad students who wanted to study the same things I did and at the beach or in the classroom, where I could make a rescue or talk to some nineteen year old, and try to make a difference in some kid's life.

In hindsight, I can see how my family was threatened by this behavior. It was different. There didn't seem to be any security in it. I must have seemed just like some old guy trying to run back to his younger, freer days. I feel bad for what they went through, but there is nothing I would change. I do not blame anyone, my family, my friends, or myself. Acceptance comes in its own time, never announced, never predicted. You don't recognize it until it is pointed out years later by someone who has earned the right to tell you that you've made it to the other side.

Mirror, Mirror

"You have to vanquish your own anonymity. You have to lose it all and win back your self by rediscovering that self through a combination of personal introspection and enlightening others."

—Anonymous

Self-identity is a common theme in the study of loss, transition, and athlete retirement, a study that includes the loss of identity and the resulting emotional trauma. When I was first experiencing some of these symptoms, I could not decipher the message, break the code, figure out why the hell I felt so freaky. Even after throwing myself into the daunting task of understanding it, answers were not coming quick enough for my taste. After nine months of various level breakthroughs that would come only in occasional fits and spurts, I finally got over the stigma that I carried about seeking "professional help." Yep, I'd go see a career counselor, a psychologist type supposedly experienced in working with former athletes. I didn't know it then, but it was all part of the submitting, the letting go.

I figured I go see this guy, have him give me some ideas and be on my way before I had to face the societal stigma of having "been to a shrink." It was completely naïve thinking but for some reason, at that point I was confusing letting go with giving up, asking for help with the inability to help myself. It wasn't so much classic machismo as it was immaturity.

When I went to my first appointment I wore a hat down low over my eyes, begging that no one would see me. And as I walked into the waiting room the first person I saw was a local newscaster and long time acquaintance who was there doing a story on one of the other counselors.

My stomach turned and the reality of my vulnerability came racing down my brain like an avalanche. There were things I could do that would make others shake their heads in awe, fearless acts beyond reproach. And there were other aspects of my being that were stuck in the shell of a scared fifteen-year-old kid.

I turned around and walked out before the lady recognized me, stood in the hallway, took a deep breath and reminded myself that I had never run away from the honest self, never cared what others thought of me so long as it was the real me. When I went back into the waiting room she was gone. And now I was a patient in need, just a bit better for the first day experience.

By my fourth visit I was hooked. I'd walk into his office and say something like, "I was just having a look at this article "Disorders of the Self and Their Treatment" by Kohut and Wolf from the *International Journal of Psychoanalysis*, and I wanted to run these ideas on the psychopathology of the fragmented self by you."

He'd look at me, laugh, and say, "What did I say about letting go of your obsessive-compulsive tendencies?" Well, I'd agree, sometimes. I'd tell him I wasn't getting enough idealized transference for my money, but I always left feeling better. In hindsight, it was because I could trust his honesty, insight, and knowledge and his ability to guide me in discovering a new self. Could I have done that on my own with only the help of a few friends and a pile of books? Of course. But it would have taken longer and I would not have gained as much through the experience.

Self-identity is a very tricky thing. A lot of counselors, psychologists, and psychiatrists are not comfortable in this area. For me, it was easy—I didn't have a choice. My self-identity had been blown apart, fragmented, disconnected, and lost to all those miles running and riding up and down the Coast Highway. I was the only one who had seen myself slip over the edge. Only I knew that I had become overidentified in this sport. And that was one witness too many.

Studying self-identity, meditating on it, and writing about it was a perfect form of healing, provided I didn't obsess on it, which I came close to doing from time to time.

I found myself analyzing other retired athletes and making amateur diagnoses about their conditions, almost always with an eye on their self-identity. I was particularly intrigued by the case of Darryl Strawberry. While Strawberry possessed incredible talent, he seemed to be oddly resentful of his skills. His actions suggested that his self-destructive behavior was purposeful and that it was intended to keep him from achieving his enormous potential.

Yet, while quietly sabotaging his own career, Strawberry was helping anybody and everybody who put a hand out. And there were many. By all accounts, he was as thoughtful and generous with his wealth as any pro athlete and much more giving of his time than the average superstar.

In discussion one day, I told a friend that it appeared as if all Darryl Strawberry wanted was to be accepted as a regular guy. But how could he? He was one of the best players in Major League Baseball, playing for the New York Yankees. That is not an environment conducive to a regular-guy lifestyle. No matter how well Strawberry played, it would never be good enough. He had chosen the hero's journey and would have to go along for the ride. After a point Darryl was no longer in control of his choices or his actions. The drugs, the alcohol, the arrests all proved that. Still Strawberry was eager to please others. He just couldn't seem to make himself happy.

Ultimately it seemed to me that he was never cut out to play the part of hero, of athlete superstar. His incredible athletic skills had twisted his fate and put him in a place where he was not supposed to be, at least not without plenty of training, advice, and guidance—little of which he received. Darryl Strawberry might have been happy as a medical supply salesman or a tennis pro at a local club. Maybe I'm wrong, but it seems his occupation and his identity were polar opposites. And it nearly killed him.

Lots of athletes struggle with issues related to self-identity when their skills fade. It doesn't matter whether they are officially retired or still earning a living off their sport.

There are markers, large and small, that propagate the identity: the way people treat you, how you are introduced, the physical reminders around your house that you can't or won't let go of. I had a closet full of trophies, well over a hundred. I displayed only one or two, and these were essentially pieces of art from which I had removed the brass inscription plate. But the rest, the ones that had somehow made it home from a race, sat in four large cardboard crates in a back bedroom. They were dusty, rusted, and dated—just like me.

But something kept me from dragging them to the Goodwill or just tossing them in the trash. A lot of people had gone to a great effort to create and award these symbols of achievement. It wouldn't be right not to pay that forward somehow.

So I took them to a big event in Central California where they also held a kids' triathlon and gave them to the race director to pass out. It was very liberating; it showed me how letting go can unbind chains you don't even recognize.

Other people carry records around with them, consciously or not. Even if you want to let it go, a major record will remain a part of your identity. For a while, the record may be a nice calling card, a good ego boost when you need one, but later it's just a number. Steve Scott has held the American record for the mile since 1982. It helped him earn a good living. But he has moved beyond the record and that existence.

"I've had that record for twenty years," Steve said. "I don't really have to rely on that record for my identity anymore. It's not who I am."

It's a profound moment. A little alarm goes off in your head. Five minutes ago you were still on your way up; now you are on your way down. You've reached the apex of your physical prowess. You're one small step closer to the clubhouse than the first tee. There are athletes who even have difficulty contemplating what they will do and who they will be on their way *up*. So they don't think about leaving until they have to. Which, by then, is too late.

I have a wonderful memory of the great American long-distance runner Bill Rodgers. He and I had run in an off-road event together, and afterward Bill sat down at a table and started talking to people and signing autographs. I did the same for thirty or forty minutes, but, tired and losing patience, I excused myself and left.

When I returned for the awards ceremony nearly two hours later, Bill was still there, still in his sweaty race uniform, still shaking hands, still answering the same questions about running he has heard for nearly twenty-five years. And the guy seemed to be enjoying himself.

A few years later, I called him up and we talked about the things in sport that define us.

"Bill, you've been at this for a long time. I know you've had to take a few breaks from running. And I know how much you love it. What was it like, you know, not being able to run?"

"Well, I went through some problems sleeping, and I was still trying to go to some races, even when I was injured. It was like, 'What the hell is going on here?' I just wasn't able to cope with it, really. That was a tricky thing. This was back around '88 or '89 or something. I had that injury for a year and a half…I remember a few times when I was really struggling with insomnia, and I think it was eating away at me mentally. And that was a tough thing—it's not a minor thing, but you can't complain. It won't do any good."

"Did you feel like the sport had overidentified you as a person?"

"I guess I never thought of my whole self as a runner. It's just what I did, what I was."

"Did it surprise you when you had some emotional difficulty with that layoff?"

"Yeah—it kind of came out of the blue. I think I need this running as a way to keep myself on an even keel, it's so important to me. It's not really the competition or the races. But I think it's the running itself, and maybe I always connected to it that way. I may do more of that down the road."

More of what? I wondered. But I couldn't ask because the answer belonged to Bill Rodgers and Bill Rodgers alone. He could run to keep sane or to make himself happy or to feed his family or because it is just what he has always done. Bill could run for any reason you could think of. But the only reason he wouldn't run would be because something out of his control prevented him. He reminded me of a spiritual leader deeply devoted to his belief. And every runner who has done a 5K or a marathon over the past twenty-five years is part of his ministry. When Boston Billy runs or talks to his flock about running, he does so with grace and symmetry because he is doing what he was born to do. I cannot picture the running community without Billy Rodgers.

I once read that insanity is simply the inability to express yourself. This seemed, at first, an oversimplification of a whole class of disorders. But as I considered this, it began to make sense. The fastest way to cause people to lose their minds is to lock them up in isolation, without any way of expressing themselves.

I looked at other transitioning athletes and asked them how they had returned to a normal life. There was no one answer of course, but the common denominator was that they had found something to believe in again, a way to express their feelings and emotions.

I reread my own notes from when I was in transition:

June 20, 1999—I feel different. It is as if there is a melding of two people inside me: the old one, whose feelings I have trouble remembering, and the new one, who is still unsure how to feel. I am not so troubled with the anxiety of not knowing who I am anymore, for I have begun to rationalize my feelings as a great and powerful transition...painful at times but worth it in the end. I hope in the end I have the courage to become exactly who I am.

I had been so busy *doing* things that I had stopped *being* anything. In my effort to keep going at breakneck speed, I was becoming more a human doing than a human being. I had to slow down and let myself just *be* for a while.

Of course, if you have ever tried to sit still and just *be*, to let existence wash over you like a wave, then you know that at first you lose your identity. Before, you were defined by what you had accomplished, who you associated with, what you did. Now none of that matters. You are trying to exist without all the attachments of life that can confuse us and remove us from our true nature.

It's not uncommon to read about movie stars and rock musicians who say that going to prison saved their lives. They were forced to sit still and do nothing, to just be. And the nature of their former lives became clear.

July 7, 1999—I try to relax and visualize how I see myself, but my consciousness is so ingrained in the old professional athlete mode that it will take some time to retrain the thinking patterns. The feelings of void are still there and very uncomfortable at times. But I understand them better and have learned to cope. At times I can sense that my ego is searching for its old self, like it doesn't quite recognize the new person, like a body that is considering rejecting a liver transplant.

I was rejecting my past. And I knew that wasn't healthy. It had given me so much. It was like rejecting my parents.

"I owe sport a great deal," the sportswriter Grantland Rice once said. "Not only has it enabled me to earn a comfortable living; it helped me to grow up."

I didn't want to seem cynical or unappreciative of what sport had given me, but I knew I had to get away from it to let a new self emerge. The problem was that I still had sponsorship contracts—I still had to race to pay the bills and keep food on the table. So I had to redefine my relationship with the sport, which basically meant I had to redefine my relationship with myself, my self-image.

I didn't *see* myself as a pro triathlete anymore. I didn't see myself as a casual competitor yet. I didn't want to race at all, because I had no motivation to beat anyone. There was no anger, no ego, no desire for the tangible rewards. I was absolutely noncompetitive. That state of mind is not conducive to winning races.

But I found some motivation in my loyalty to the sponsors and race directors who had been so supportive over the years. I would do my best and not think too much about it.

It's amazing where you can find motivation and, ultimately, a sense of identity. I remember when the disabled athlete Paul Martin, a national record holder in the half marathon and the 5K for lower-leg amputees, as well as a two-time national cycling champion, told me that he had been a mediocre athlete until he had lost his leg. In losing that leg, in challenging himself to be one of the best disabled athletes in the world, he had found an identity in the absence of a body part. One thinks of Nietzsche: "He who has a why to live for, can bear almost any how."

Or Viktor Frankl. Frankl spent World War II in a Nazi death camp. A Jewish psychotherapist and creator of a form of therapy he called Logotherapy, Frankl came to understand self-identity as a form of finding meaning in one's life. In his landmark text, *Man's Search for Meaning*, Frankl cited a survey in which social scientists from Johns Hopkins University had asked nearly eight thousand students at forty-eight colleges what they considered "very important." Sixteen percent said "making a lot of money." But a full 78% said their first goal was "finding a purpose and meaning to my life."

"Of course, there may be some cases," added Frankl, "in which an individual's concern of values is really a camouflage of hidden inner conflicts."

When a person experiences any major transition in life, his or her values may change. There are any number of anecdotes detailing people's near-death experiences and their sudden subsequent return to values based in family, health, religion, spirituality, or personal fulfillment. But we never know if the inner conflicts buried beneath that shift are addressed. I am reminded of the statistics showing an increase in the divorce rate for married couples who have been divorced before. The new marriage may cover over inner conflicts or personality traits that doomed the first; you need to address these, or you'll just drag your old baggage into the next relationship.

Even if an athlete's time in sport was a dream come true, any past-due nightmares will come to collect. When the NFL quarterback Joe Montana was given his farewell party upon retirement, he told the assembled masses in San Francisco that playing pro football had been his dream.

"The unfortunate thing about my dream," Montana said, "is you end up waking up. This is like a wake-up call for me." And when you wake up in the morning, you aren't always who you were in your dreams.

An ex-player of Montana's stature will have many opportunities to find meaning and purpose in life. When I finally caught up with him via cell phone as he rode a New York City taxi, he spoke of competing on cutting horses. He seemed enthusiastic, almost excited about this new venture.

But for every superstar like Joe Montana, there are dozens of journeyman players who aren't so worried about finding their true selves as finding a paycheck. And their identity usually conforms to their occupation. Mark Collins, a member of the New York Giants Super Bowl XXV championship team, once told a reporter for the *San Diego Union-Tribune*, "I'm no longer a football player. I'm a man trying to make a living."

Or take the case of Ickey Woods, of the infamous "Ickey Shuffle." Woods led the league in rushing yards per carry one year and would perform his creative dance routine after each of the fifteen touchdowns he scored. By 1992 he was retired with two bad knees and was selling meat door to door. "I do what I gotta do, brother," he told the press. "I've got babies to feed. The first two years, I couldn't accept it being over," he recalls. "After that, when nobody was calling, I realized it was over. There is a life after football."

Yes, there is life after everything, even death if you believe in the concept. And when you get to that other side, you are rarely the same person you were. From what I have seen, you are a better person, more caring, more mature, with the ability to put things in perspective, even the hellish period that you may have gone through while you existed between jobs, between worlds, between identities. But you do it because your other choice is to lie down and die a slow, pathetic death. There are enough stories of athletes who have ended up homeless, athletes who are addicted to drugs and alcohol, living sad, sad lives for reasons that make even a cynical fan want to go find that athlete, take him in, give him another chance. For that should not be his identity—that should not be the identity of any unfortunate soul who fell on hard times and just kept falling.

Where Do They End Up?

*"Safety, entitlement, power...those are all fantasies. We
don't drive our destinies. Not in that way."*

—Jim MacLaren

"*W*here will I end up?"
To answer the question properly, you must know
where you've been. And that's not as simple as it seems.
I don't know too many people who can sit down and retrace their
lives with any great detail. They might have the places and dates correct, some of the names, and most of the big events that mark the
edges—births, graduations, marriages, more births, tragedies, victories, new jobs, illnesses, and deaths—it's not that hard to take a few
photos, jot down the date, and tuck them away in the album in the upstairs closet.

But to be able to recall how you felt at those times, what you
were thinking about, what thoughts and emotions ran through that
head of yours when you threw your graduation cap high into a blue
afternoon sky? Were you happy when you bought that first house?
Sad when the divorce was finalized? Relieved that you were fired, or
shocked that one of your family members could be taken from this
earth?

Our brains control those feelings and emotions. Too painful?
Repress it. Too powerful? Make it dull. Too joyous? Forget it in the
endless search to find it again. But if we can hold onto those feelings,
we can begin to know where we've been, what we've experienced,
and what our lives have meant. And that will guide us in what is left
of our years on earth.

Some people are better at remembering than others. Children remember well. Their minds haven't yet developed the capacity to filter. Spiritual people, especially those trained in some of the Eastern philosophies such as Zen meditation and mindfulness, remember feelings. Certain occupations foster feelings so powerful that it's hard *not* to remember. Healers and caregivers, even when surrounded by tragedy, remember well. I worked in a hospital emergency room only for a short period, but I can tell you the color of the drapes and the names of my favorite nurses almost twenty-five years later. And I can remember exactly how I felt when I saw a bullet hole in a man's head for the first time.

Career mothers are like that too. The truly selfless moms, the ones who don't know the meaning of the word "me," can tell you exactly how scared they were when their first daughter went off to college or when their son received his draft notice.

Soldiers remember. Those who have seen battle remember things they wish they could forget, horrifying images of death and mayhem. But they can also feel the brotherhood of the men, the thrill of the firefight, and the incomparable joy of simply being alive after other men have tried in vain to kill you.

Lifelong athletes have the opportunity to experience unbridled emotion, something that seems lacking in our world today. They know that too much feeling at the wrong time can hurt a performance, but sometimes the emotion is too strong to ignore. They can't help but sing, laugh, cry, and swear—all in a single inning, or a single lap of the track. Why do you think golf has become such a popular sport? Do you think millions of people around the world actually enjoy the activity of chasing a little white ball around a lawn? Of course not. Golf makes you feel things. In a few hours you can run the gamut of emotions, from incredulous wonder to bottom-feeding disgust. Golf, in all its polyester glory, makes people feel alive.

Now, take that human potential for deep emotion and stretch it out over a protracted period. Imagine hurting like hell in training, day in and day out, but having a group of fellow athletes to help you make it through. Imagine ten years of running, almost always by yourself, ten years of hill repeats and three-hour long runs, when not a day goes by that your legs don't ache. But when you're out in front, moving swiftly, effortlessly, over the final hundred yards, and the crowd is screaming but you don't hear them, and your toes are bleeding but you don't feel them, and as the finish line comes up against your chest, and hands you do not know are holding you up, slapping you on the back, touching you because you have something they want—that is a moment so raw and free that what you feel erases every pounding step of the past ten years. At that moment, you know exactly why you sacrificed, what your purpose is, and who you are.

That is one of the draws of an athlete's life—it can teach you who you are at that period in life. Things can become very clear in battle. As Anna Freud once said, "War cures all neuroses."

But when that opportunity for clarity and the single-minded sense of purpose goes away, when the wars are over, where does the athlete turn to replace what he or she has lost?

The answer is everywhere and nowhere. They go in search of that lost group of friends and the pure success of winning a race. They go in search of the feelings that their previous life once gave them. They are drawn back to the thing that gave them so much. And if they can't get it in one sport, they might try another.

Alberto Salazar went from running marathons to winning one of the most famous ultramarathons in the world, the Comrades Marathon near Durban, South Africa, a fifty-four-mile race that attracts 15,000 competitors. And he won it on his first try.

Motocross champion Johnny O'Mara tried mountain biking after he left the motorized version behind and was immediately successful in the pro ranks. Fellow motocross champion Jeff Ward finished third at the Indianapolis 500, and then backed up that performance with a near win two years later. Olympic speed skater Eric Heiden "dabbled" in professional cycling while he waited to enter medical school and was picked up as a rider by one of America's best teams. Michael Jordan played baseball, Greg LeMond raced cars, Herschel Walker was the brakeman for an Olympic bobsled team. Sometimes the public can't quite figure it out. I mean, how dare these athletes change roles?

But no matter what the fans have invested in the athlete's role as a player, they have no investment in his or her post-playing days as a human being. We may treat athletic celebrities like royalty, but like kings and queens throughout history, they are disposed of quickly when they fail to serve their purpose.

At some point in life, most people have a kingdom of sorts. It might be their job, their family, their neighborhood, their friends, or their material wealth. It is something they have worked for, something they have a right to, something important to them; it might even define them.

Take it away and what happens next is a timeless story. The king or queen goes off in search of a new domain. For athletes, the search usually begins when they walk away from the playing field. It should begin while they are playing their best years. And their journey ends when everyone's journey ends—when they have taken their last breath.

If you have the means, you can run a racing team, buy real estate, hell, buy the major league team you once played for and name yourself manager. Those dreams are reserved for the franchise players who made a lot of money and invested it wisely, who are smart, who have always been smart with their careers.

Why does Michael Jordan continue to beat the odds while Wilt Chamberlain dies at sixty-three years old, or Walter Payton at forty-five, or Dave McNally at sixty? How is it that some feel the scalding of the past without even knowing the source while others use the flame for warmth and light?

What twist in fate allows Cal Ripken, Jr. the opportunity to develop new ballparks and youth leagues all over the country, while a guy like Jackie Jensen—the only athlete ever to play in the Rose Bowl, the World Series, and the Major League Baseball All Star Game—dies of a heart attack at fifty-five?

Jensen, an incredibly talented multisport athlete before there was such a label, was an All-American fullback at the University of California, Los Angeles in the late 1940s and the American League MVP in 1958 as a Boston Red Sox outfielder. His life beyond sport was rife with tragedy and disappointment. A fear of flying compromised his career as a ball player; he and his wife (a former Olympic diver) divorced; he lost his job as the coach at Cal Berkley; and he suffered ongoing health problems. All these things wove a tale of pathos.

In 1959, one year before he would sit out the entire season rather than spend another year away from his family, Jensen coauthored an article in the *Saturday Evening Post* entitled, "My Ambition Is to Quit." In the article Jensen said, "It takes a certain breed of guy to be happy with a ballplayer's day-to-day existence. I'm not the type...If I were consumed with a passion for the game, as many men are, I suppose I couldn't be happy away from it...Maybe I wasn't meant to be a big-league ballplayer. I have the soul of a floorwalker."

Eric Heiden becomes a successful orthopedic surgeon, John McEnroe is a well-respected TV commentator, and Rod Milburn, Olympic gold medalist in the 110-meter hurdles, is found dead in a railcar full of a bleach solution at the paper mill where he worked. The Associated Press article read: "There was no indication of how Milburn, forty-seven, wound up in the car at the Georgia Pacific plant near Baton Rouge." Authorities said they did not suspect foul play. There was little information on the accident, the implications left only to the reader and those who knew of Milburn's great career and his return to the lifestyle of a man just doing his job, getting by.

No one really suspected anything more than an accident.

And why should they? Who knows what was going through Milburn's mind at the time. By all accounts, he was well-adjusted and caring—in the words of Southern College track coach Johnny Thomas, "a really good guy."

Many people die too young. Others seem to die too old. The decision is not ours to make.

I cannot begin to say specifically why some athletes do well after sport and others do not. I have completed one of the most exhaustive qualitative research projects on the subject to date, I have written hundreds of pages, and my best answer is that much of it depends on how you perceive yourself. If you can only see yourself as a professional athlete—or as a fireman or a soldier or a scientist or a tree trimmer or a child—then the day will probably come when you no longer have that occupation as an identity, and you will not be able to see yourself at all. And, at least for a while, the harder you look, the further you disappear into the fog.

But no matter whether you're an athlete, a housewife, a truck driver, or the king of a small country, when your reign is over and you're lost in yourself, you must weather the storm. Because someday you will come back, not to the same house or the same field, but you will come home to some feeling of completeness. And you will smile, not knowing exactly why. It's not like a fading migraine or the pain of a toothache, which falls away like ice chipped from a windshield. It's more like high cirrus clouds that thin as the sun heats the earth and the earth warms the sky.

One day your patience is rewarded and your smile deepens and you tell yourself you're going to be all right. Whoever the hell you are, you'll be just fine.

The Circle Game

"I was telling writers I thought I had me only three or four years left, but I wasn't believing it anymore. I was feeling like I could go on forever."
                                    —Satchel Paige, *Maybe I'll Pitch Forever*

*I*t's been four years since I won a race. It's been five years, maybe six, since I walked away from a broken neck that might have made me another athlete who died before his name. It's been just over a year since I had a big portion of my nose cut off due to skin cancer, and twelve months since I wrote the first few words of this book. If I look very closely, I can still see tiny bloodstains down between the keys.

I count twenty-five years since my first triathlon, twenty since I taught a sailing class, twenty-two since I put a needle in the arm of a guy who had been shot in the head, twelve since I tried to start an IV on myself the night before the Ironman in an attempt to "pre-hydrate," two days since I last waxed nostalgic with a friend about the good old days, the vicissitudes of growing old, and tactics for keeping our kids out of the same trouble we so desperately sought when we were their age. And it's been twenty minutes since I could write a sentence that wouldn't fall off the page with melodrama, nostalgia, and a sappy longing for those times when our conscience was clear, our faces were smooth, and the future was any god damned thing we wanted it to be.

Most of the time I'm okay; I've dealt with it. And I take great joy and fulfillment in helping those who struggle with the passing years. It's the best therapy I've found. But other times, when I'm on my own and some outside stimulus sneaks in the back door and wiggles its forgotten little head into my own, I go all the way back. I am like an alcoholic, but my addiction is to the devil-may-care vibrancy of youth. Why? I don't know, but as Pascal said, "The heart has its own reason which reason does not know."

Some days I imagine myself standing in front of a like-minded and eclectic group at some local hotel. It's a meeting for Youth Anonymous. The room would be called the California Suite or something similar. There in the front row is Dakota. His name used to be Bud, and he has a long ponytail and deep-set eyes that are green and knowing. He says that he plays in an alternative rock band. But mostly they play '70s covers like Boston and Cheap Trick. Lately, they've had trouble getting gigs. He won't tell me his age. Only the most confident in this group will.

Next to him is Lauren. She tells everybody she is a poet. They all know her from the "open mike" nights around town. While she waits for a book contract, she is a checkout girl at Von's Market. I might guess her age as forty-two, or thirty-eight with extra eyeliner and that black pullover she wears. But this group doesn't "do" that age thing. No. That's why they're here. Lauren's poetry would be good. It would have an edgy, raw feel to it. I'd buy the book.

I see myself standing up in front of the group and reciting the Youth Anonymous Creed, "Hi, my name is Scott Tinley and I love everything associated with youth." But then, if the thoughts were flowing and the words could keep up, I would say this:

"Well, fuck that. The media are trying to convince me to buy products that make me look and feel young. Some of my friends, well, they've bought into the sale. They say, 'You just gotta try it.' Others seem to be old before their time, having given up on health, the past, that vibrancy and innocence I seek. And in doing so, they have given up on the future. They seem dead to me. Their funeral started a long time ago. But the body remains above ground.

"Yeah, folks, I'm thirty-eight, or forty-two, or forty-six—what the hell difference does it make? I have a lot of miles on my body. But I haven't given up. And *that's* what puts people underground before they need to be."

Then I would pause to look around and notice that a few people had gotten up to leave but others were leaning forward, as if not quite sure whether to shake their heads in pity or nod them in agreement. And I would continue, seeking purchase in the eyes of those who might understand, or at least not misunderstand.

"I loved my job, but I realize now that while part of it was a brilliant quest, other parts were babbling illusion. I pursued it with all I had, but I was also pulled forward by something I didn't. Professional sport is a game, part hide-and-seek, part Life, part Monopoly. It is real when the athlete does something positive with his or her fame. It is real when they screw up and do something stupid with their fame. It is real when the ball is in play and the dancers are on the ice and the wheels are humming and the athlete is exposing human potential in all its beauty and courage. But a lot of it is not real. If you want constant, unrelenting reality, go to a homeless shelter or a veterans' hospital. If you want youth, don't let anybody take away your innocence. And if you want sport, go coach a kids' team at the YMCA."

Easy for you to say, the audience would snicker. You got to live it. Looking good makes me feel good. What an ungrateful bastard! So who made you lord of life transition anyway?

Every barb would have some truth to it. But if I had enough courage, I would stand up and answer them.

"It absorbed me, inhabited me, and the return made me stronger. But I do not consider myself a victim and I do not speak lightly about one of the best things that happened to me, and one of the most difficult. As one patient said, 'I am thankful for my beautiful neuroses.' Sport at any level can bend time and allow the athlete to enter that intervening space where senses pop and life has a heightened quality. People join softball leagues and learn tai chi and rent little sailboats on Sunday afternoons because sport takes them out of the tedium of mediocrity, if only for a few hours. Professional or weekend warrior— it's the same. Both begin and end somewhere in the middle, different for having denied the mundane, the unchallenged elements of each waking hour."

I have returned to the middle but will forever disavow anything medium. Seeing my daughter get dressed up for her first formal dance is as good as winning a national championship. Watching my wife's wide, wide smile when she catches a good wave on a body board, or hearing my son play "Heart and Soul" on the piano for the eighty-fifth time—I am learning that these too are victories of great significance, ones that beat with time, in time, not against it. I would never again dream of raising my arms in victory as I cross the finish line.

I know now that in many ways I will never again reach that same pinnacle of the human experience I found in sport, when I possessed the freedom and will to move swiftly over land and water with no one but myself to guide, to incite, or to blame. But I will gain contentment with and from others.

I have learned that dreams are not only a picture of our wishes and a review of our past, but also a glimpse at our future—should we dare to risk it all once again and chase them into a sun closer to falling than rising.

When it appears that our dreams have ended and we are subject to a futureless future, our dreams will begin again. When we are lucky enough to hit bottom, we will have something to push off of. Count yourself lucky if you never suffer. Count yourself luckier if you do.

Take off your dress shoes, rub your toes in the warm sand, and let the tide take you back out so that you can go forward with a new clarity of purpose and intent, and with the lighted laughter of a child.

When we are pulled from our mother's womb, under a bank of hospital lights, amid instruments and harried voices and frenetic activity, what must our first thoughts be? "The hell with this shit! It's cold and crazy out here. Who are all these faces and what do they want with me? Hey man, put me back. That was nice and warm in there."

But we gradually accept our place in the world. And we become separate from the world around us and the people who have created us as we grow into our own selves. That is the ultimate form of acceptance: allowing ourselves to become who we are, as the poet would say, "in a world that is trying its hardest to prevent that from happening."

One night, well past midnight, an e-mail from an old friend arrived. He'd known me, watched me succeed and fail, rise and fall through the passing seasons:

"You realized your wildest dreams, and now realize that they have left you empty. I have studied this problem as both observer and participant for years. Your wife and family will never understand. Don't expect them to. It's a lonely journey, the journey of truth that Nietzsche's Zarathustra and Socrates describe. But books don't give answers; they give clues to help you cope, to make you realize that you're not alone in the endless endeavor to find answers to shifting-sand questions."

Nobody had spoken to me like this in the past. I hadn't earned this wisdom. I hadn't suffered enough, so the words would have been wasted on me. Now I drank like a thirsty man.

I got up, put on a coat, and walked the empty streets of my small beach town until just before sunrise. When I came back the house was quiet and still, and I realized that my past life in sport had been both a road to self-knowledge and a dead-end escape; I learned things about myself and who I was in sport, but I never unmasked indelible truths. Sport had allowed me to gloss over the parts of my past that were painful and submerged, like a deep splinter that gradually works its way out. It was more fun than I can ever tell. And it was over.

I watched the sun come up, drank coffee, and waited for something to happen. In a single night I had forfeited blood membership in a community that I will always love. No matter how hard I might try after that night, I could never again pretend to be part of the family of athletes.

Sitting in my den, I looked around the room and saw for the first time things that had been there for months. An old, tattered black-and-white photo of my dad pole-vaulting back in high school; the frame was made of bamboo, same as the pole he used. I had memorized his best height: twelve feet, six inches. Back then, before foam, they landed in pits filled with wood shavings. Below was a picture of a man walking down a railroad line with a guitar strapped to his back, and then a picture of my daughter when she was four, and a family Christmas card when we all looked so happy it hurt. On the shelf was a copy of Kafka's *The Metamorphosis*; right next to that was Nicosia's epic *Home to War* and John Knowles's *A Separate Peace*. There was a box of incense, fingernail clippers, a shell from some cold, lonely beach way up north, a candle, a tape recorder, a stack of overdue bills, a tide table from the year before, and one little glass race trophy missing its brass plate. I was trying to let my past go by digging it up, and all around me were exhumed signposts telling me how to go forward by going backward.

But right there, between the tape measure and the expired coupons for a yoga class, was a little spring, probably from a flashlight that had come apart. I picked up the spring and turned it in my fingers. Bits and pieces were falling away from my past like fall leaves. I looked at the spring and realized that life is not so much a circle as a spring that winds back onto itself with every revolution. And with each turn, you move a little farther toward the end.

I walked my son to school and stood in line to play handball with him and the others. The kids seemed bigger that day. I couldn't get them out easily. The bell rang. I went to give my son a hug; even though I knew he might be embarrassed by it, I needed it. And he knew I did.

"Hey pops," he called out as I walked off the playground.

"Yeah Dane?"

"You should go get in the ocean. It makes you feel better."

"You think?"

"Yeah Dad. Go surfing. Love ya, bye." And in a moment he had taught me more than Nietzsche and Campbell and the others.

My nine-year-old son was daring me to be myself in a world that was trying its hardest to make me anything but. And he was showing me that giving what you had to give was about all you needed to do. The rest would take care of itself.

I rode down to the beach and asked my friend Pat, the lifeguard chief in Del Mar, if he needed any help. He stared at me for a moment, trying to decide if I was joking. But he had seen it before—the ocean, the rescues, the camaraderie, it gets in your blood. I needed something red and pure to keep that warrior's heart beating; some need to be needed, to be who I was, to give what I could.

"Yeah, sure. We could use an old dog around here. Dig out your crusty red trunks and come in on Saturday. You remember how to swim don't you?"

Ironman Redux

So the years spin by and now the boy is twenty
Though his dreams have lost some grandeur coming true
There'll be new dreams, maybe better dreams and plenty
Before the last revolving year is through
　　　　　　　　　　—Joni Mitchell, "The Circle Game"

I opened a letter yesterday from the organizers of the Ironman World Championship. They were inviting me to compete in the twenty-fifth anniversary event in 2003. Suddenly it was 1999 and I was back at the awards banquet of the last Ironman I had competed in, sitting on a sidewalk curb next to Jimmy Riccetello, gnawing on chicken bones, and half listening to what was happening up on the stage two hundred yards away.

"Hey S. T., check it out, they're talking about that car you're gonna win."

Isuzu Motors was a title sponsor that year, and part of their deal was to award a new car to a person who had shown tenacity and commitment to the event.

"Dude, they got to give you that car, man. They know you ain't gonna be coming back again. How else are they gonna pay you back for twenty straight years of kicking your ass out there? A gold watch? Listen, they're talking about who deserves it and stuff. That's YOU man! Hey, you gonna upgrade to the leather interior?"

"Jimmy, you're on drugs. I'm not getting any car. Besides, I already have a car. And it runs pretty good if it doesn't get too hot."

"No, man. I'm serious. They're talking about it right now. Get real. This race and the corporation behind it is worth something. Your

knees and hips are no better than my twelve-year-old dog Rudy's.
Who else are they going to give the car to? I say forget the leather and
get four-wheel drive."

"I'll bet you $20 they give it to some lady with a passel of kids
who needs it more than me."

"Deal. They owe you something bro. This event became valuable
on the backs of real people, giving real performances."

"Naw. I got what I came for. And it wasn't any new car."

"What if it was something cool, like a guitar or that '61 Chevy
Impala you've been talking about all these years?"

"A good guitar? Like a Taylor twelve-string?"

"Ah, you see? You ain't such an idealist after all. Take the car and
sell it. Go find that old Chevy you want and be *over* this place."

I was over it, had been for a while. No regrets, just well...*over* it.
Looking at the letter I wondered if I could go back, and in what capacity. I didn't want to be a prop, sitting in a corner signing autographs, regaling the fans with stories of my glory days. But I had
accepted my new role and would enjoy reconnecting with the many
friends who had also invested in the 2,880 miles I had competed in
Hawaii over twenty races (each race was a total of 140 miles: a 2.4-
mile swim, a 112-mile bike, and a 26-mile run). What I had done, I had
not done alone.

I thought that I could probably watch the race and cheer others on.
Yes, I could do that now. Then I felt like maybe I could actually participate in the event, even without the time to train for it properly—just
rely on muscle memory to carry me over the 3,000-mile mark. But
would that be smart? Hadn't I grown out of this? Or had I grown into
some different kind of competitor? One who needs only to finish?
Finish what though? Where I was headed there was no finish line.

And when I finished writing this book, I still didn't know if I
would compete; so much like the words themselves, sometimes clear,
other times just my stream of consciousness trying to figure it out.

I had trained hard for the race in 1999; I wanted to give a good
showing as a sort of tribute to all those who had supported me over
the years. My goal was a top-twenty finish, even though I was twenty

years older than many of my competitors. Instead, I spent the day wallowing in the middle, caught by two flat tires, two flat legs, and a bowing of the arch that had always pushed me down a notch in the standings with each passing year. I witnessed the event from the inside out, a place where the everyman finds his limits. I had strangers stop in the middle of their race and offer a spare tire, a word of encouragement, a piece of their spirit. They didn't do it because I was a former champion. They gave of themselves because it defined their own sense of competition, which is to say, their victory was in the participation. I was never more proud of my peers.

Somehow I felt like I owed them something. I had been losing commitment for success over the years, and along with it, respect for the event. I didn't like the feeling, but couldn't seem to avoid its ugly draw. The year before, in 1998, the race organizers had initiated computerized timing. At various points along the course, receiver strips would pick up signals from the chips competitors wore and transmit each athlete's time and position to the media center, the webcast, and out to the world. I had a hard time with technology creeping into something that had been sacred to me so, being the jerk that I could be, I took the chip off my ankle and hid it inside a saddle bag on the lead motorcycle. For a while, hundreds of thousands of fans logged onto the Internet site believed that number twenty-eight, the forty-year-old former champion Tinley, was leading the race. I made up some lame excuse that it had fallen off in the swim start area and one of the camera crew must have picked it up and forgotten about it. Twisted as it was, I still think it was one of the best practical jokes of my career. Not everyone agreed.

The race in 1999 was no joke. When I finally finished the bike ride, climbed off, and waddled over to put on my running shoes, something dark and dangerous clouded over me and I had a feeling of impending doom. My heart felt like it would jump out of my chest and I became short of breath. The world got small, and the noise and confusion sounded like devil's laughter. I was scared.

I asked someone to call over my friend Dr. P. Z. Pearce, who was working in the medical tent.

"P. Z., something is terribly wrong with me. I don't know if I can do this."

Dr. Pearce didn't tell me the truth; he knew better than to say that I was staring down the barrel of a loaded gun called *change*. How could he explain the pathophysiology of a panic attack when I was supposed to put on my damn running shoes and charge out onto the course, just as I had in nineteen previous races? But I also knew that I couldn't just kill time, as Thoreau said, "without injuring eternity."

"Listen S. T., you're probably just a little dehydrated. Sit here for a second, relax, and if you want to call it a day that's fine. You've left enough blood on this island for one lifetime. You'll be fine."

He was right: I would be fine. But because of all the people like him, I needed to finish. So I changed shoes, shook his hand, said nothing, and ran.

I reread the 2003 invitation, "We cordially invite you...," and felt my heart rate go up a beat or two. That's one thing I will carry around with me from my career as an endurance athlete: I can sense minor changes in my body, almost as if I have an internal monitor plugged into my vital signs. There are times, though, when I wish I was more aware of *why* I feel the way I do.

This one wasn't hard to figure out. I was being asked to come back, to relive so many highs and lows of my career, to be put on display, but also to give something back. I just wasn't sure yet.

At mile five of the marathon in 1999, my last marathon, that wonderfully hideous final leg of the Ironman, my legs started to loosen up. And so did my attitude. I ran by a yard full of well-wishers, as full of *looking good*s and *go get 'em*s as they were of afternoon mai tais. One girl handed me a flower, which I stuck in my hat. A quarter mile later somebody yelled, "Nice flower bruddah!" So for the next four miles, I stopped and picked the best flower of each kind I thought might look good in my rapidly expanding Hawaiian headdress. By the time I hit the turnaround point I smelled like a florist, and was beginning to run like one too.

The last few miles I broke down and wept my way through the crowds, salty tears mixing with every past step of joy and pain, streaming down from behind my sunglasses onto the pavement where it had all started long ago when I was half my age. I was done.

The next night at the awards, I finished my chicken bone, got up from the curb, collected my $20 bet from Jimmy, and went home to pack my bike.

And by the time you read this, I will have ether competed in one more race, or not. Either way, it won't matter. It was what it was.

Game Over?

"As the physically weak man can make himself strong by careful and patient training, so the man of weak thoughts can make them strong by exercising himself in right thinking."

—James Allen

*I*n November 2002, Manute Bol, the seven-foot, seven-inch, 225-pound former NBA shot blocker, agreed to play for the Indianapolis Ice in the Central Hockey League. He was forty at the time and had recently beat former NFL player William "The Refrigerator" Perry in Fox TV's Celebrity Boxing show.

Bol, born in southern Sudan, has spent most of his life savings trying to bring peace to his war-torn country. The general manager of the Ice, Larry Linde, said, "We're always looking for a unique angle. We like to expose our fans to people they might like to meet."

On February 1, 2003, Michael Jordan, who would turn forty a few weeks later, scored forty-five points to lead his Washington Wizards to a 109–104 victory over the New Orleans Hornets.

"Everybody talks about his age and everything," said Jamal Mashburn of the Hornets. "The guy can still play. You don't get 30,000 points without knowing how to play."

Not a month earlier, Milton Javier Flores, the starting goalkeeper for the Honduran national soccer team, was shot six times as he sat in his parked car. The twenty-eight-year-old known as "Chocolate" died later that day in the city of San Pedro Sula.

Nearly six weeks before that, Patrick Ewing, one of basketball's greatest players, announced his retirement. Although he is a virtual

shoo-in for the Hall of Fame, there was no ceremonial news confer-
ence or parade. His illustrious career spanning seventeen seasons
seemed to have already been forgotten.

"It's time to move on," said Ewing. "It was a great ride...I'm at
peace."

In actual playing time, top athletes don't get much face-to-face competition. On the track, the mile is run in less than four minutes, and
the 10K in twenty-seven—about the same as a TV sitcom, including
commercials. A baseball game is longer, but there sure seems to be a
lot of standing around. Football takes place in quick, violent spurts;
a basketball game involves several miles of running, but they take
timeouts and substitute players. Swimming races are won and lost by
a fingernail.

The only sure thing is that sooner or later the game or the race will
end. There will be other games with other players. Some will have
long, prosperous careers; some will be journeyman players who are
happy to see a few minutes of playing time here or there. Some will
sign for more money than their parents earned in a lifetime and then
get injured in the first and only season they play. Some will make just
enough to keep them in new running shoes and a small apartment,
chasing that dancing carrot, dreaming that fame and fortune are just
a lucky break away.

The faces look the same in joyous victory and heartbreaking defeat. The faces look the same under helmets, hats, and goggles. Only
the names change. And always there will be a story worth telling in
sport, always a film at 11:00. Ironically, the faster you go, the sooner
you get to the finish line. And when you get there and catch your
breath, you wonder where the time went and you want to do it all
over again. But speed has a cost, as does everything. One of those
costs is the perpetuation of the illusion of youth. Keep running kid,
you'll never grow old.

I used to laugh at the guys who refused to exercise saying, "The
body only has so many heartbeats—I don't want to waste them running around in damn circles." Of course, they were wrong. Now it

appears that a certain amount of exercise can prolong a life, but too much can shorten it. How much is too much? How should I know? I'm still alive.

Sport gives life and sport can take it away. Jesse Billauer was one of the best surfers in the Malibu area of Southern California. A well-liked seventeen-year-old, he dreamed of a future on the professional circuit. Two months after I broke my neck in the mountain bike accident and walked away from it, Jesse broke his when he hit the sandy bottom on a small-wave day at Zuma Beach, north of his Malibu home.

Six years later I met Jesse out surfing near my home in Del Mar. Now he rides waves lying on a specially built surfboard, maneuvering it with what little control he has over the muscles in his upper torso. Jesse broke C-6, the same bone I did, the same as Christopher Reeve. The two of them will live out their lives in wheelchairs, at least until someone comes up with a way to rebuild spinal cords.

Jesse Billauer lives every day to the fullest. He is one of those rare individuals who has found triumph in tragedy, no different from Reeve, David Bailey, Bill Johnson, or a thousand others who will remain in the shadows, living out their lives the best way they know how. They do it because they are sportsmen first. They knew the risks and they knew the rewards. They played the game as best they could. No one can say if their lives are better or worse, really. They are different for the tragedy, but they are human still. They did not choose this challenge, it chose them, for the same reason it passed me by.

They use the skills they learned in sport to go about the business of living a full and rewarding life. They have a life after sport when they are closer to physical death than many people who walk around with normal bodies. They know that in the end, there is no end...just another type of game to play.

One day I went out to an old motocross track near where we used to ride as kids, before the stucco jungle subdivisions and Ford Explorers replaced the oak- and sage-laden coastal valleys of Southern California. I was there to watch my old friend David Bailey coach future motocross champions, his sixteen-year-old son Sean included. Of course, I brought one of my ancient machines, not to feel left out, and plodded along tentatively while the fearless kids lapped me.

Taking a break, I watched Bailey, who sat in his wheelchair and hollered at them from the edge of the track, "No, no. You gotta want it! You gotta keep that speed UP through the jumps."

His protégés didn't look over at David and think, "Look where it got you?" Not a one. They think, as I do, of how much courage and inner confidence it must take to pass on his knowledge. In effect David is telling his students, "Do as I did and you'll be a national champion like I was. Do as I did and you could end up in chair like I did." In the end, the lesson that David Bailey would offer his students, in words and example, is one of informed choice.

Jeff Emig, a successful rider who came after Bailey, had to make a choice. Seeing David in his chair helped him make it.

"I was on my fourth lap of a practice session on May 4th," Jeff recalls, "just doing some engine testing. And then the throttle stuck wide open for a second leading up to a small tabletop jump. I hit it wide open in third gear, over-jumped it big time, and separated from the bike in the air. I landed without the bike and compressed my body into the ground, compound fracturing my right tibula-fibula and crushing the second lumbar vertebrae.

"At first I didn't feel my legs and I was thinking that I was paralyzed, lying facedown in the mud thinking 'Wow, this is what it feels like.'"

Or doesn't feel like, you might think. You are in that purgatory where some force, maybe God if you believe, is deciding whether you would better serve your purpose on earth paralyzed or able-bodied. And in that netherworld where you exist, a moment ago a top athlete and a moment from now perhaps paralyzed, your mind does funny things. Jim MacLaren knows this well.

"After my second accident when I was hit by that truck during the race, I was laying in the back of the ambulance," he recalls, "and I couldn't feel my legs and my arms were strapped down, I thought well, maybe I'm *only* a paraplegic and I can go and break the world record for the marathon in a wheelchair. I was in that pure race mode. In my mind I was still an athlete with great potential."

Was Jim in denial? Of course, but even with a severed spinal cord that would leave him without the use of his legs and just enough use of his arms to keep him in a sensual and tactile purgatory for the rest of his life, his mind was moving forward to the next challenge. Jim MacLaren, the athlete, was trying to shake off the devils that chased his soul while the wail of the ambulance's siren raced him away.

For Jeff Emig, the story was different. You can't say that he and I were luckier than MacLaren or Bailey; we just weren't chosen to end up with the same physical challenges at that period in our lives.

"Eventually," says Emig, "I felt the pain from my broken leg, then I moved my left one. I totally knew that I broke my back, though, my entire midsection was tightened up…It was at that point that I said to myself, 'This is it. I do not want to have to make a comeback. I'm retiring.'"

"I am lucky that I can still ride and enjoy the sport I love so much," he concludes. "Others aren't."

Luck. What about luck? Is anybody who gets to play a sport professionally lucky? Are guys who bust their necks but get up and walk away lucky? Is luck what happens, as the cliché goes, when "preparation meets opportunity"?

No. Luck is like a child's kaleidoscope: The colors and consequences that come through it depend on how much light you let into the tube.

Jim MacLaren feels he is a lucky man because he has some use of his arms and, on a good day, a bit of sensation in his legs. He feels he is lucky because his injuries have given him an extraordinary life, a life full of searching and pain and enlightenment and humility and despair and a kind of peace in knowing that, as hard as it is to grasp, he was born to live wounded. If he were a regular, able-bodied person, he would not be able to do what he was born to do—to inspire people with his courage and his insight.

"I feel like I finally have all the knowledge that I need to do the clearing out of the past for myself," MacLaren says. "I might get hit with another brick but I know that I can set myself free because I'm not attached to things that don't matter. I won't be denied freedom for myself."

Athletes exercise a great deal of control over their lives, which is one reason why the lifestyle is so attractive. There is less duplicity and ambiguity in athletics than in other professions. I knew early on I couldn't exist for any length of time in the business world. Not because I felt intimidated or I strongly disliked many aspects of it; I simply found that I was happier having control over my days and my environment than I was working for someone else. Later I found that this sense of control is partly an illusion: some things we control and others control us.

The Pulitzer Prize-winning author Katherine Anne Porter once said that salvation can only be found through religion and art. I believe that great feats of physical endurance include traits of both.

A few weeks ago, I attended the annual endurance sports awards. It's a celebration of sorts, of past accomplishments by runners, cyclists, swimmers, triathletes—by athletes who compete by themselves for every imaginable reason.

I had been going to this same function, held in various forms, for eighteen years. Some years I had been given great honors, such as athlete of the year or induction into some hall of fame, but this year I was going to celebrate the others and see some old friends.

Midway through the evening I was standing in the back of the giant hall that contained close to five hundred athletes, media people, and family, and a new feeling came over me, a feeling I mostly welcomed, although it carried a hint of sadness.

I knew that if I ever was to step on that stage again, it would be for something that happened in the past, in a former life. Nobody in this crowd was going to give me an award for being a great teacher or a writer or a father or a husband. And then I realized what a wonderfully unique slice of life these people represented. Indeed, there were present more than a few world record holders, Olympians, and men and women who had been the best in the world at what they had done.

The second half of this junior epiphany was the cold, harsh, but not exactly uncomfortable realization that we were all facing the same challenges—no, that's too good a word—the same *shit* that life slings out at every man, woman, and dog.

As I ambled over to the bar for another beer, I could bear witness to various undiagnosed medical problems and more than a few friends in therapy for depression, anxiety, and that great psychological catch-all, "nondescript neuroses." There were young men with the beginnings of osteoarthritis and women having affairs that everybody knew would get back to their husbands; there were child-athletes with prostheses and wheelchair athletes who had more feeling in their hearts than the fifty pairs of able-bodied shaved legs tucked under the ornate banquet tables topped with traditional rubber-chicken dinners. There were a few absences, men and women who had been standing at that same bar next to me two or four or six years ago. They were dead. But the only place I heard their names was in the silent echo of a missed friend.

All around the room were people who had been affected by something called life. They were the chosen, the best at what they did, but that fact was no shield against the slings and arrows of bill collectors and cancer cells and sick kids and deadlines and receding hairlines and the little hairs that start to grow in your ears. They had lived the exposed life, as does anybody who takes one step beyond what is asked. There was a certain repetitive music to the pathos, but I didn't really hear it until I entered my own breath. Strangely, I didn't feel sorry for them, just a part of them. At first, it was comforting in a twisted sort of way. Then, as the night unfolded the elements of human drama, not the rehashed hyperbole of film clips, came the acknowledgement that these athletes were special people, as are taxi drivers, grocery clerks, and finish carpenters; and there was an untwisting of the wires that had snagged my essential freedom. For the first time I came to know these people I had raced for twenty-five years.

I walked to the bathroom and splashed cold water on my face, and when I looked in the mirror, a man introduced himself to me. He had my face, my smile, my sadness, my past. And in his eyes he had my hope. And that was enough. I had made my way back. Now it was time to move on.

Yeah, I had and would continue to have my share of obstacles, but who the hell hasn't? It's life, baby. And I was fucking glad to be a part of it.

My friends Paul Huddle and Roch Frey walked up to the bar.

"Two beers on him," they said, not missing a beat. I would've done the same. It was a form of mutual respect.

Roch and Paul, who are coaches and consultants in the sport of triathlon, had just finished a four-day camp for athletes from all over the country. They were beat.

In the morning they would grab an extra half hour of sleep and then head to the office to start working on training programs for their clients. It seemed like a fun job. But it was hard work.

Roch downed his beer quickly and ordered another. Turning to the both of us, he began the lament of a man at the crossroads who might be searching but might be satisfied. "Man, this is getting tough, I'm tired of it," he said in half-jest. "What are we going to do when we grow up?"

Huddle, ever the levelheaded pragmatist, looked at Roch with a sneer and then motioned to the next award recipient about to take the stage. We knew him as one of America's greatest cyclists, as did many of those in the room.

Davis Phinney got on stage and began his tale of life after sport. The room was still. His hands shook as if he were very nervous, but that wasn't the case. He told the crowd that they should be very appreciative of the little things in life.

"If your toast comes up and it's not burnt," he said, "raise your arms and say, YES!"

And as he raised his arms, the father, husband, motivational speaker, and cycling legend almost fell over backward. He grabbed for the podium, nearly knocking over the trophy he was about to receive while the twin microphones shook like toy spaceman antennae. A few people covered their mouths and there was an uncomfortable silence in the room felt by everybody—everybody but Phinney. He laughed at himself and told the crowd his nerves were shattered.

Two "handlers" came up to help him but he had steadied himself by then. "Let me get through this," he told them, "just give me a minute, one moment please."

"I welcome this challenge," he told the crowd. And in the next sixty seconds Phinney revealed that he was suffering from Parkinson's disease, said he was doing pretty good, he was doing all right. Then he stepped away from the podium, took a deep breath, and raised his arms in a huge victory salute. This time he was as steady as the days when he used to raise those same arms while sprinting to victory at thirty miles per hour. For the moment his toast was golden brown, for the moment he was doing just fine, thank you.

And as tears fell on the dark green carpet, Paul turned to Roch and me and whispered, "In the morning we're going to get up, watch our feet move when we ask them to, our hands hold still when we type. We're going to appreciate our families, and go about our jobs. That's what we're going to do." I found myself silently nodding and thought, oh my God, he's telling me we are already grown up. When did that happen?

Epilogue

The morning after the awards dinner I remembered all of it, from the number of asparagus on my plate (exactly four) to the number of glasses of wine I had drank (exactly four). A few details were missing, though, like why did I come home with no shoes? And what happened to me after the last award was given out? I wasn't drunk. I was still in good shape, dammit. Heck, I would've raced anybody in the room that night. We could have pooled our asparagus and marked out a running course. But I didn't. I didn't race anybody.

After that final dinner, that Last Supper, I ceased talking about my life as an athlete. I became very good at changing the subject, at never having to put my tongue up against the truth of my past. It wasn't something that I did consciously but somehow, like weddings and birthdays and funerals, that awards dinner had marked the edge of a curve. I went home realizing that I didn't need to be there, that my presence was appreciated but not required. My final acceptance of that called for a certain muteness. And so I went into a period of self-induced amnesia.

But I did write about it—virtually nonstop for a year. I couldn't explain it, didn't even try to. I was objectifying my experience of living between lives, between identities. I was telling myself through the written word what it was like to be "depersonalized," secretly hoping that someone else would come along and say, "Yeah, it's no big deal to be a ghost. Everybody lives under a white sheet at one period in their lives."

I was invested in my neuroses. I knew that I didn't want to end up with a shadowy recollection of what it was like in that netherworld; it had been too long and too painful. It owed me something. So I wrote about it, depositing descriptions of feelings and thoughts in a paper bank, to be withdrawn at a future date, with a substantial penalty for early withdrawal.

A few nights after the banquet, I was coming home from a big day at the university. I had taught my creative writing class, spending most of the class trying to get the students to tell *me* why they wrote. Sometimes you can learn more from your students than they will ever learn from you.

I had gone to a sports psychology seminar, a detailed discussion about the intricacies of helping other athletes overcome their non-physical challenges. And I had spent several hours in the library, doing research and listening to the voices of all the great dead writers.

When the library closed I was asleep, my head on a book about the greatest boxing matches of all time. I didn't remember pulling the book off the shelf; I don't even like boxing. But I remember the dream I was having.

In my dream I was running down a long, straight trail high in the Colorado Rockies with my old friend and rival Scott Molina. The trail was lined with pine and aspen, and it seemed to converge at a point in the distance as railroad tracks do. Long periods of silence were peppered with intense laughter, and books hung from the branches instead of cones. There was a library stillness in the air. Our feet never hit the ground: they came close and then rose up again like cars on a Ferris wheel. We weren't heroes or star athletes, nor were we aging jocks trying to be something we weren't and could never be again. We were just two friends out for a run, nothing more, nothing less. That, then, was something we shared. When I awoke to the loudspeakers announcing that the library would close in ten minutes, I wondered why I had lost close contact with my best friend in the sport. It was no excuse that Molina lived halfway around the world in Christchurch, New Zealand. I was afraid that I would never again be able to run that trail, that light, that free. Scott Molina had been my fiercest competitor in the sport. We had raced each other no fewer than two hundred times, often staring across the chasm of victor and bridesmaid as we accepted our awards afterward. Somehow we had become friends through it all.

I deciphered the library dream: I missed the camaraderie and the lightness of being that comes with sport. Much of what I had been doing since retiring was trying to replace those things in some way. And I wondered if I ever would.

As I drove home that night it began to rain, a light mist growing into thick, heavy drops by the time I passed the old college pool where I used to work out. I pulled over and looked at the edge of the dark square shape, recalling the time we had pulled the cover off one morning to reveal a drowned young woman who had climbed the fence with a few other drunk students the night before and had gotten stuck under the large, tight cover as if it were polar ice. They closed the pool for two days and put up extra signs. But kids from the college still sneak in and swim on warm summer nights.

I thought about climbing the fence and doing a few laps. I'd peel back the cover and see how fast I could swim the one-hundred-yard freestyle, or how far I could swim underwater. I'd taunt death again, as I had before, light and free.

But as I stood in the black rain, shedding my own skin and slipping out of my own history, that floating feeling from my dream mixed with the past and the rain and I knew that, eventually, I would be okay. It wasn't so much a sense of peace as an absence of conflict. And in that moment, shared with the ghost of a nineteen-year-old looking for a way out, it was enough.

When is anything enough? When you are born with certain personality traits—and you can substitute "highly focused" for addictive, or "goal-driven" for obsessive-compulsive—the best you can do is recognize the traits and direct them in as healthy a direction as possible.

I can never return to my years of full-time athletics and I can never stand in the same river twice. But when I find myself trying to get two or maybe three post-graduate degrees, teaching two or three classes, working on two or three new books, well, I can stop and remind myself that all I'm doing is replacing one obsession with another—a bit healthier maybe, but not enough, as Thomas Merton once said, to "untwist the warping of my essential freedom or loose me from the devils that hung like vampires on my soul."

I think that's what I was trying to do when I turned down an opportunity to coach another athlete, and when I gave all my trophies away: I was freeing myself from the platitudes of athletic stardom and allowing my past to untwist and slowly slip away until I could bring it back and appreciate it for all that it was.

I remember talking to my friend Linda Buchanan about her life after sport. At one point in the mid 1980s, Linda was probably the best female triathlete in the world. And then she was gone, vanished from the circuit. Just like that. In a quest similar to my own, she went back to school and threw herself into leading the examined life in the hopes of understanding why she felt empty, directionless, and without purpose. I asked her how long it took until she felt "normal" again. Ten years, she told me.

It may take me ten years to feel "normal" again, or I may never feel the way I did when I was a champion athlete or when I was a young kid trying to find my way. I'd like to think that I can recapture the essence of my thoughts and emotions at those times, to remember so that I can teach my kids and my students, and myself. Sport taught me many things, and continues to do so. If I can preserve enough of its reality in my past, just enough that would remain beyond reproach to anything else around, maybe it would keep it pure for me. That would help me find the acceptance of myself and my past that I so covet. And that might help me unfold into what my true purpose is.

When I started this book nearly a year ago to the day, I was groggy from the general anesthesia that had put me out while the docs cut out the skin cancer, the sins of my youth I think I said, the cost of two decades of training under a Southern California sun.

Now as I end it, I am once again trying to shake off the fogginess of anesthesia. This time they were putting a couple of Swiss-made stainless steel screws into my left foot to fix a bone I broke while flying a lifeguard rescue boat over a large wave and landing wrong. Another cost of an occupation under the SoCal sun.

It's a hobby-job, as my wife calls it, something I do for fun. But that's not right. It's so much more. The old warrior's heart is still beating, and I still need to be needed, to do something of substance, to live and work with clarity and simplicity. When people are drowning, you go save their ass.

In twenty-five years of racing, all I had done was fracture a few bones in my neck and twist my ankle a thousand times. Never a stitch or a cast or an operation. My injuries, broken neck included, were Nietzscheian speed bumps: They slowed me down and pissed me off, but they never killed me, they only made me stronger.

Now my year has begun and ended under the knife, cutting here, screwing there. I wasn't cracking those jokes about how sex, drugs, and rock and roll had become ear, nose, and throat, but these auguries of mortality were changing me. My feelings of loss and confusion were only a ploy to season my mood and prepare me for the metamorphosis. I needed to be comfortable in the darkness, striving. I needed to accept change and turmoil, death and rebirth. And mostly I needed to learn the final stage of loss—acceptance.

When my wife dropped me off for my foot operation, I seemed calm. I was looking forward to reading some books. There were a few races coming up over the next months, but if I had to pull out, nobody would sue me and we wouldn't be sleeping in the car. I was supposed to be retired anyway. The waves in the spring are typically windy and blown out, I told myself. A few weeks downtime to write or paint or help the kids with their homework would do me good. There are no accidents, I finally convinced myself. Everything happens for a reason.

When the nurse took my blood pressure it was high. I was putting up a good front but the numbers don't lie. I was nervous, maybe even scared. What if something went wrong and I couldn't ever run again? I was retreating into my narcissistic self; I was too concerned with the body when I should have been focusing on the mind, or even the soul.

The doctor doing the surgery made some joke about me being more of an Ironman now because I would truly have metal parts inside me. He was thirty-two years old, in fifth grade when I won my first Ironman. I smiled, took some deep breaths, and remembered how certain Zen masters could will themselves to stop bleeding from an open wound. I added yoga to my list of things I wanted to become proficient at in the next year. Yeah, I could do it in a year.

But a year is a long time, and ten years is even longer. Better that I take it a month, no, a week, no, a day, no—better I accept my place right here and now. Make the best of it. Relax, breathe in, breathe out. Slow down and let the past catch up with me. Quit running away from it, since I won't be able to run for a few months anyway. I did some great things in my life as an athlete. Yeah, it was a hell of a good life.

Acknowledgments

Those who made this book possible are as many and varied as the thoughts and emotions that ran through my mind in its creation. They came from infields, the end zones and the ends of the earth. And within the pages, they came to stay, though barely long enough for my hands to write their stories and lives. While this book is framed around my journey out of sport and off the sports pages, it is more a collective tale, a co-op of camaraderie among many. It could not and would not have been done without the dozens of selfless individuals willing to offer of themselves, their dreams and tragedies, successes, and failures.

At the risk of leaving someone out, I will not attempt to list every athlete, editor, and friend. If you find your name in this book, I offer my sincerest appreciation and gratitude for contributing directly or indirectly to this body of work. If any reader finds but a snippet of guidance, it is because of your willingness to share. However, it must be noted that the entire project could not have come to fruition without the likes of those who work in the business of publishing. To that end, several people should be noted: My old friend Bill Katovsky for putting a pen in my hand, getting a publisher on the phone, and for refusing to let me move onto other writing projects until I told this story, all the folks at The Lyons Press having faith in this project, especially Tom McCarthy. What a joy to work with someone who knows words, knows sport, and knows people.

I need to thank all my writerly peers at SDSU, the instructors, the students; I am fortunate to count them as teachers and friends.

Finally, my children Torrie and Dane, who allowed me to get my homework done first before helping them with theirs; what a gift they are.